KETO, THE DELICIOUS ROAD TO HEALTH & FITNESS

In this book "Keto, The delicious road to health & fitness" you will find delicious & healthy keto recipes which will help you maintain your fitness and health goals in a very different and delicious way, Maintaining health was never this easy that you eat delicious food and maintain your health.

A word on KETO :

Keto diet is one of the most popular and known as most effective diet now a days,

In keto diet we lose fat by lowering carbs ratio and increasing good fat ratio in our diet.

The diet "works" when you are able to achieve ketosis. The claimed benefits of ketosis are numerous:

Lose weight quickly;

Slow down the onset of hunger pangs;

Stabilize the energy level during the day;

Decrease the symptoms of epilepsy;

What are gifts of KETO:

Very high consumption of lipids (75% of intakes)

Unchanged protein intake

Considerable reduction in carbohydrate intake

Causes unpleasant symptoms in the first few weeks (ketogenic flu)

Rapid weight loss

The state of ketosis would have many health benefits (energy boost, protection against certain pathologies, etc.)

How this book is so helpful?

This book is so helpful for those who are on KETO diet,

This book will keep them on track by not let them eat same food again and again,

This book is offering a wide range of KETO recipes so that you can experience new recipes with exciting tastes every day and you can lose your weight while enjoying it.

Table of contents

KETO BREAD

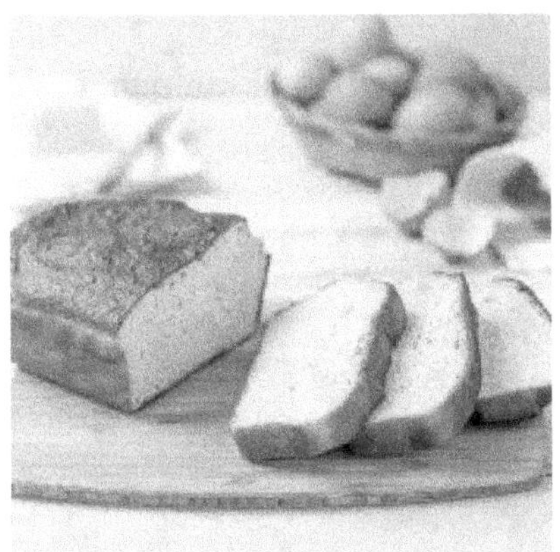

Ingredients:

7 eggs

5,3 oz (150 g) of flax seeds, ground into flour

1,8 oz (50 g) sesame seeds (optional)

7,9 oz (225 g)ground almonds

3 tsp olive oil

1 tsp salted coffee

1 sachet of sifted baking powder

0,05 gal (200 ml) spring water

The preparation:

- Mix: flax flour, ground almonds, salt & sifted yeast

- Add sesame seeds (or other), eggs & mix

-   Add the water, the oil & mix ... The dough is elastic
    and flexible

-   Pour into the baking pan lined with baking paper,
    smooth the top

Put in the oven for 35 minutes at 392 ° F (200 ° C).

NAPOLITAN KETOGENIC

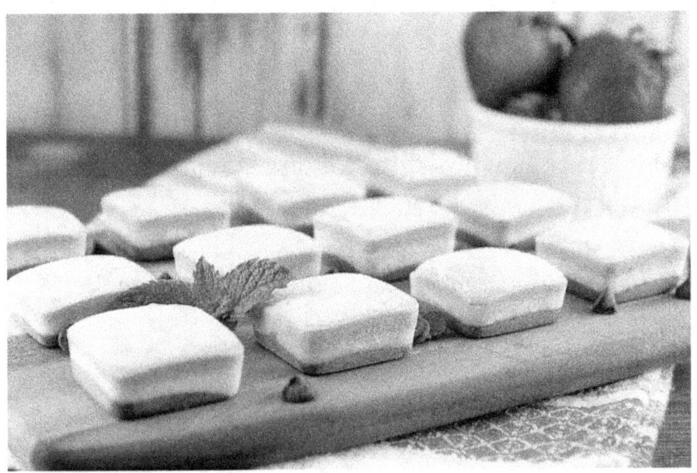

Ingredients:

4 eggs

7,1 oz (200 g) of butter

2,8 oz (80 g) coconut flour

2,5 oz (70 g) erythritol

¼ tsp liquid stevia or other sweeteners

1,8 oz (50 g) of 100% dark chocolate

1 sachet of baking powder or 1 tsp of baking soda

For the chocolate frosting:

1,1 oz (30 g) of 100% dark chocolate

¼ tsp liquid stevia or other sweeteners

The preparation:

Bowl 1:

- Melt the butter

- Mix the eggs with erythritol and stevia until this mixture turns white

- Add coconut flour, yeast & mix. Pour the melted butter & mix

Bowl 2:

- Melt the 1,8 oz (50 g) of chocolate

- put 1/3 of the dough from bowl 1 in bowl 2, add the chocolate & mix

Bowl 3:

- Melt the 1,1 oz (30 g) of chocolate, add 1 tsp liquid stevia or other sweeteners & mix

- Pour bowl 3 into a mold → pour bowl 2 over it → pour bowl 1 on top

Bake at 356 ° F (180 ° C) for about 15 minutes.

SAUTÉED PORK WITH BRUSCHETTA

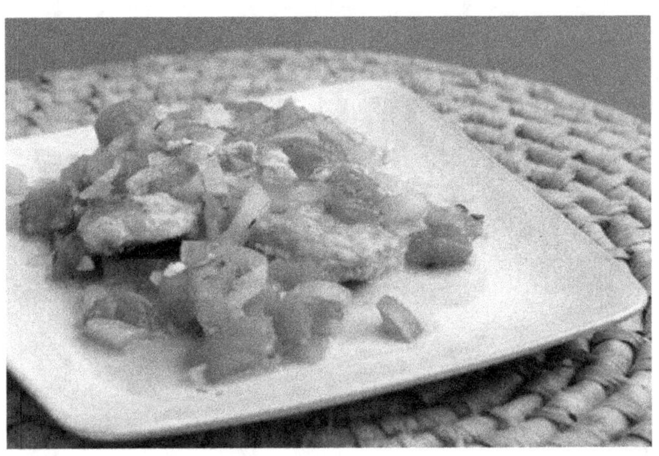

Ingredients:

21,2 oz (600 g) pork tenderloin/chicken

1 zucchini cut in half rounds

1 container of 12 oz (340 g) bruschetta

0,016 gal (60 ml) balsamic vinaigrette

0,016 gal (60 ml) minced fresh basil

The preparation:

- Cut the pork tenderloin/chicken into strips

- Heat a little olive oil in a large skillet. Cook the

- pork strips for 1 to 2 minutes on each side

-	Add the zucchini to the pan and cook for another 1 to 2 minutes (if your pan isn't big enough take another one)

-	Add the bruschetta and balsamic vinaigrette (in another pan). Bring to a boil, then simmer everything for 2 to 3 minutes over low heat

-	When ready to serve, garnish with basil and salt and pepper

MARINARA DUMPLINGS

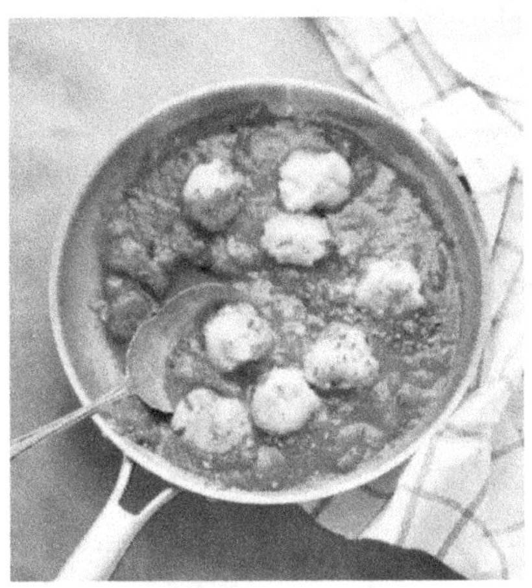

Ingredients:

0,13 gal (500 ml) marinara sauce

15,9 oz (450 g) of dumplings, about 24 dumplings store-bought

0,10 gal (375 ml) grated mozzarella cheese

2 tbs (30 ml) chopped fresh parsley

The preparation:

- Mix the marinara sauce with the dumplings in a heated frying pan.

- Cover with grated mozzarella and sprinkle with parsley

Cook for 12 to 15 minutes

NACHO SALSA, CHEESE AND SAUSAGE

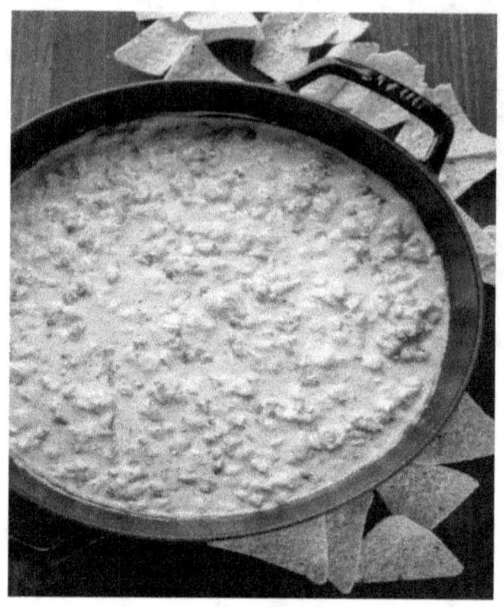

Ingredients:

1 bag of 7,9 oz (225 g) corn chips

4 Italian sausages cooked and cut into rings

0,10 gal (375 ml) salsa

0,13 gal (500 ml) shredded tex-mex cheese mix

The preparation:

- Preheat the oven to 400 ° F (205 ° C)

- Divide the corn chips on an aluminum tray or in a cast iron skillet

-   Garnish with slices of Italian sausage and salsa. Sprinkle with grated cheese.

-   Bake 8 to 10 minutes, until cheese is melted

-   Keep the nacho warm on the propane fireplace, previously heated over low heat

TRIO COLD MEAT WRAPS

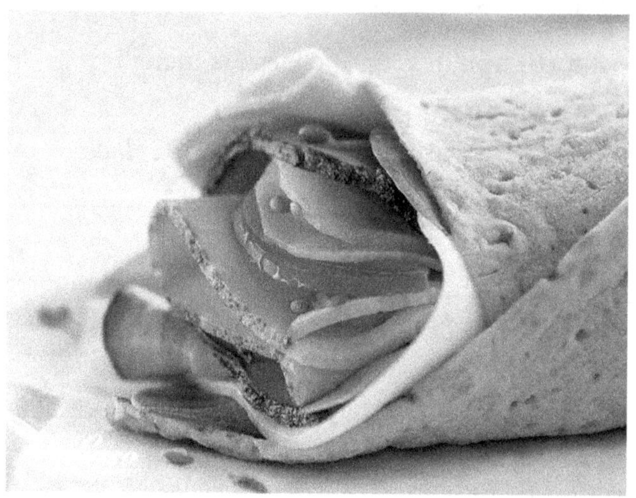

Ingredients:

8 medium tortillas

8 Boston lettuce leaves

1 red pepper cut into sticks

8 slices of ham

8 slices of turkey

16 slices of salami

For the mustard sauce:

2 tbs Dijon mustard

1 tbs Old-fashioned mustard

1 tbs Honey

The preparation:

- Mix the Dijon mustard with the old-fashioned mustard and honey

- Brush the tortillas with the mustard mixture

- Spread Boston lettuce, red pepper sticks, ham slices, turkey slices and salami slices over the tortillas

- Roll the tortillas tightly and enjoy!

STRAWBERRY-YOGURT POPSICLES

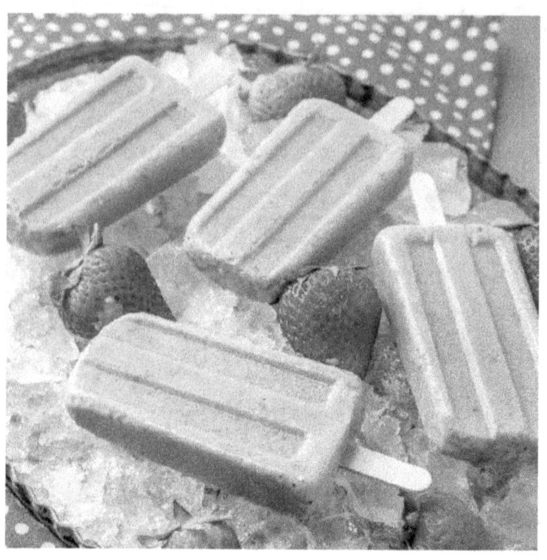

Ingredients:

12 to 18 small strawberries

15,9 oz (450 g) strawberries

0,13 gal (500 ml) vanilla Greek yogurt

0,016 gal (60 ml) maple syrup

The preparation:

- Cut the strawberries into small pieces and set aside in the freezer

- Mix the rest of the ingredients 1 minute, until a smooth texture is obtained

-    Add the pieces of strawberries and stir with a spoon

-    Divide the preparation among the popsicle molds.
     Put a popsicle stick in the center of each popsicle

Place in the freezer for 3 to 4 hours, until the popsicles are
well frozen.

WHIPPED RICOTTA RADISH

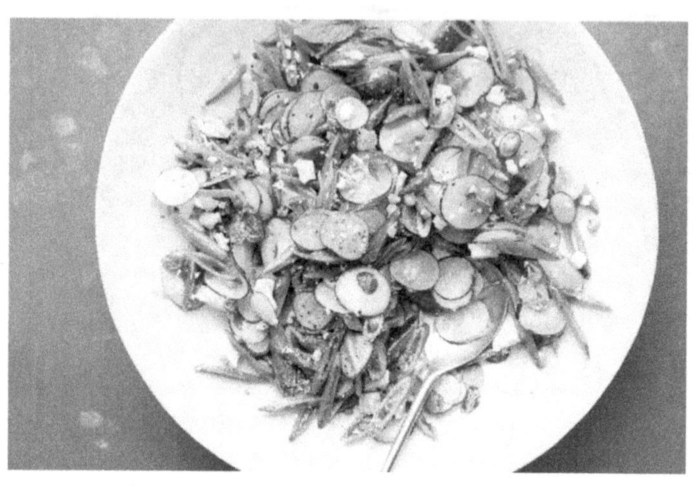

Ingredients:

Radish 20

½ lemon

Ricotta cheese 5% 10,6 oz (300 g)

1 tbs (15 ml) olive oil

Pepper and salt

2 tbs (30 ml) fresh herbs (see preparation)

Freshly ground pepper

The preparation:

- Cut the radishes in slices

- Get a bowl and squeeze the half lemon, add the ricotta, the olive oil, generous amount of pepper & pinch of salt. Mix 1 minute

- Spread it out on a large serving plate and divide the radishes over the ricotta. Garnish with fresh herbs, a drizzle of olive oil, crushed pepper and a pinch of fleur de sel

- Serve with pita breads or crackers

SPREAD WITH HERBS AND OLIVE OIL

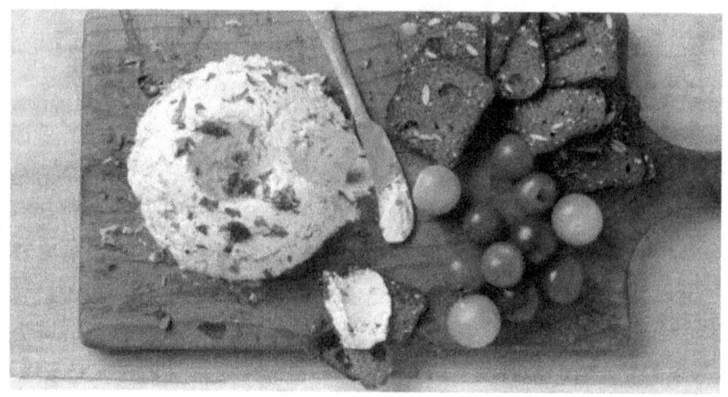

Ingredients:

3 tbs (45 ml) fresh herbs

10,6 oz (300 g) soft ripened goat cheese

3 tbs (45) ml olive oil

¼ tsp (1 ml) hot pepper flakes

Freshly ground pepper

The preparation:

- Finely chop the herbs

- Put 1/3 of the goat cheese in a glass jar with a capacity of approximately 0,13 gal (500 ml)

- Add 1 tbs (15 ml) of oil, 1 tbs (15 ml) of herbs & pinch of hot pepper flakes. Garnish with crushed pepper

Repeat with the rest of the ingredients to get three floors

- Serve with toast

DUKKA WITH PISTACHIOS AND ALMONDS

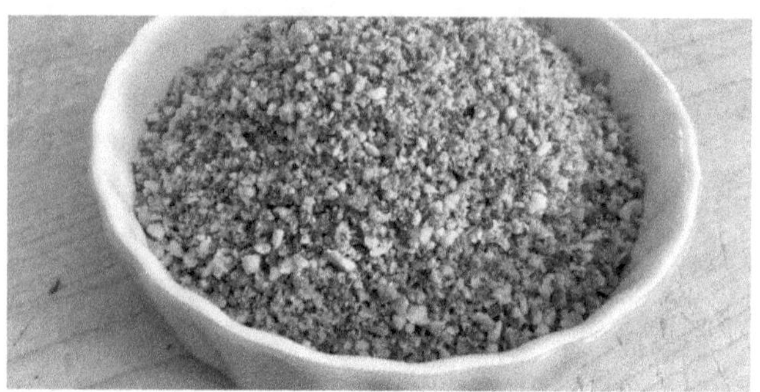

Ingredients:

Natural pistachios 6 tbs (90 ml)

Natural almonds 6 tbs (90 ml)

Fennel seeds 1 tbs (15 ml)

Mustard seeds 1 tbs (15 ml)

¼ tsp (1 ml) salt

The preparation:

- Brown the nuts, fennel seeds and mustard seeds for
  2 minutes in a non-stick skillet preheated over
  medium-high heat, without adding any fat
  - o Stir occasionally

- Crush the nuts and spices with a knife on a cutting
  board. Put it in a small bowl and mix with some salt

- Serve with pitas and olive oil

KETO TORTILLAS

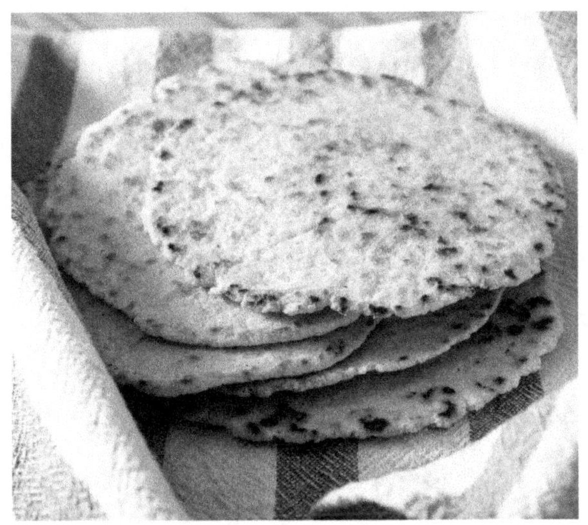

Ingredients:

4,6 oz (130 g) coconut flour

4 tbs powdered psyllium

4,4 oz (125 g) of butter or coconut oil

1/4 tsp of garlic powder

1/4 tsp cumin

1/2 tsp pepper

1/4 tsp salt (optional)

The preparation:

- Melt the butter and set it aside

-   Mix the coconut flour, psyllium, spices, salt and the melted butter in a bowl

-   You can use some hot water to bind the dough well

-   Separate the dough into 8 balls (each about 91 g)

-   Heat a pancake pan (put a little oil in it), if your pan does not stick, there is no point in oiling.

-   Flatten the balls (between two parchment paper) and cook over a not too high heat and let them slowly take on color, turning them from time to time

CELERY VELOUTE RAVE

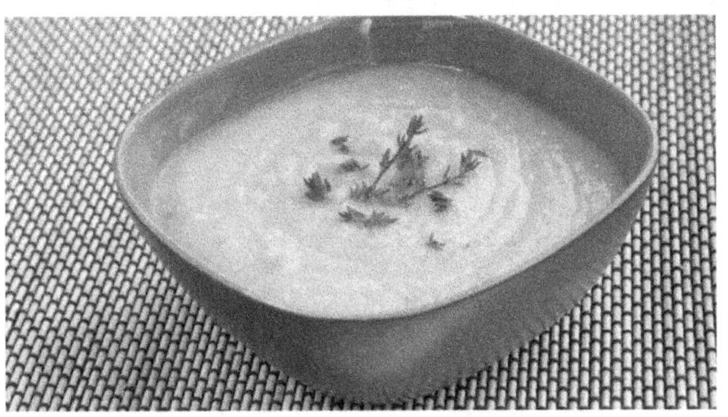

Ingredients:

10,6 oz (300 g) peeled celeriac

7,1 oz (200 g) coconut milk

1,8 oz (50g) of butter

½ tsp of turmeric

6 scallops

Salt, pepper and other spices of your choice

The preparation:

-   Cook the pieces of celeriac with the coconut milk

-   Melt 1,1 oz (30 g) of butter in a saucepan and add
    the turmeric & the celeriac cooked in coconut milk.
    Mix everything

-   Brown the scallops for 1 minute on each side in a hot pan with the rest of the butter

-   Serve with celery cream, garnish with a few cilantro leaves

PORK RILLETTES KETO CAKE

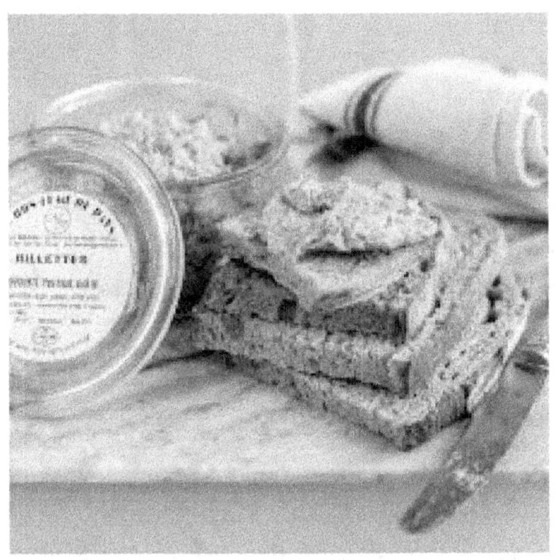

Ingredients:

0,88 oz (25 g) coconut oil

0,88 oz (25 g) ghee

5,3 oz (150 g) pork rillettes

3 eggs

2,8 oz (80 g) of coconut flour I use this one with less carbohydrates

6,5 oz (185 g) coconut milk

½ tsp baking soda or ½ sachet baking powder

Chives parsley or coriander at will

Salt, pepper or chili or whatever you want more

The preparation:

- Put all the dry ingredients and the herbs and spices in a bowl

- In another bowl: beat the eggs into an omelet, add the coconut oil and the melted ghee together (you can replace it with: butter, only ghee or only coconut oil) and add the coconut milk, continue beating

- Add the rillettes, mix again, and finally add the dry ingredients.

- bake for 25 to 30 minutes (when the cake is golden brown) in an oven previously heated to 356 ° F (180 ° C)

KETO SALTED CAKE

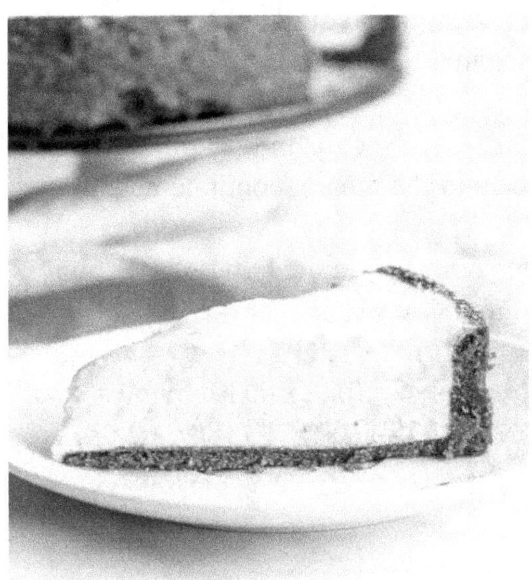

Ingredients:

4,1 oz (115 g) small grated zucchini

1,8 oz (50 g) ghee or butter or coconut oil

6,3 (180 g) pork rillettes

4 small or 3 large eggs

1,8 oz (50 g) of coconut flour

5,6 oz (160 g) liquid cream

½ tsp baking soda or ½ sachet baking powder

Chives parsley or coriander at will

Salt, pepper or chili

The preparation:

- Put the grated zucchini and all the dry ingredients, herbs and spices in a bowl

- In another bowl: beat the eggs into an omelet, add the melted ghee and the cream, continue beating

- Add the rillettes & mix, add the bowl of zucchini with the dry ingredients & mix

- Put it in a mold and bake for 25 to 30 minutes in an oven previously heated to 356 ° F (180 ° C)

COCONUT FLOUR KETO ROLLS

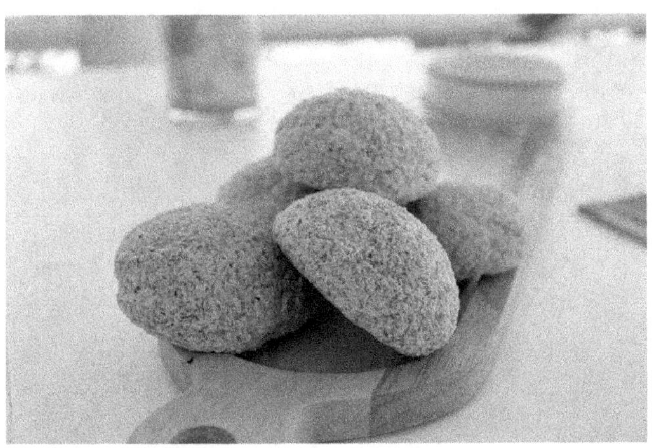

Ingredients:

3,5 oz (100 g) of coconut flour

0,7 oz (20 g) blond psyllium

2,1 oz (60 g) butter

2 eggs

¼ tsp cumin

¼ tsp garlic powder or garlic and herbs

½ tsp apple cider vinegar (optional)

½ tsp baking powder or baking powder

The preparation:

- Preheat the oven to 356 ° F (180 ° C)

- Melt the butter

- Put all the dry ingredients in a bowl and mix. Add the melted butter, the vinegar and the two eggs & mix

- Then gradually pour in some hot water and mix until it forms a ball

- Separate this ball into 6 small ones and put them on a baking sheet, covered with baking paper

Bake for about 1 hour in the oven.

LEMON CURD KETO COOKIE

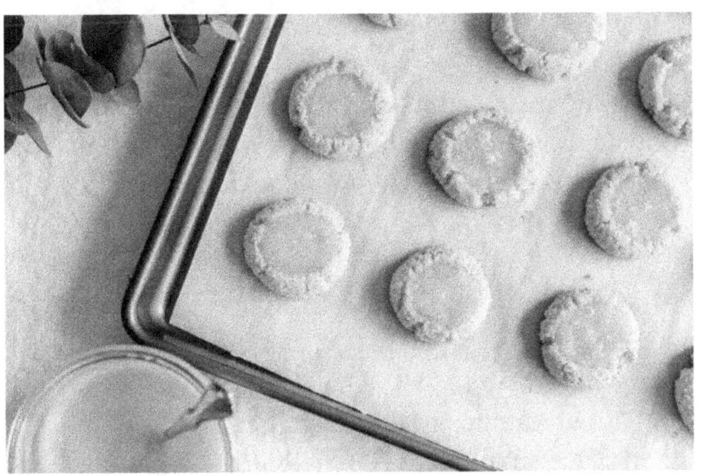

Ingredients:

3,5 oz (100 g) macadamia nuts

1,8 oz (50 g) butter

1,4 oz (40 g) almond flour or almond powder

0,88 oz (25 g) grated coconut

0,7 oz (20 g) coconut flour

1/4 tsp stevia

1/4 tsp baking soda

1 pinch of cinnamon

The preparation:

- Take out the butter in advance to soften it

- Press the macadamia nuts and turn them into powder and add coconut oil to get paste. The more paste you want the more oil you need, so it's to your liking

- Mix all the dry ingredients in a bowl, add the butter and knead, you will get a shortcrust pastry

- Put a few minutes in the fridge to freeze the butter, then place small pieces of the dough on baking paper or in a cookie mold (see picture)

- make a small hole in the middle and garnish with what you want (jam, chocolate, etc ...)

- Bake at 356 ° F (180 ° C) for about 15 minutes, as soon as they are golden, they are ready.

LEMON KETO MERINGUE PIE

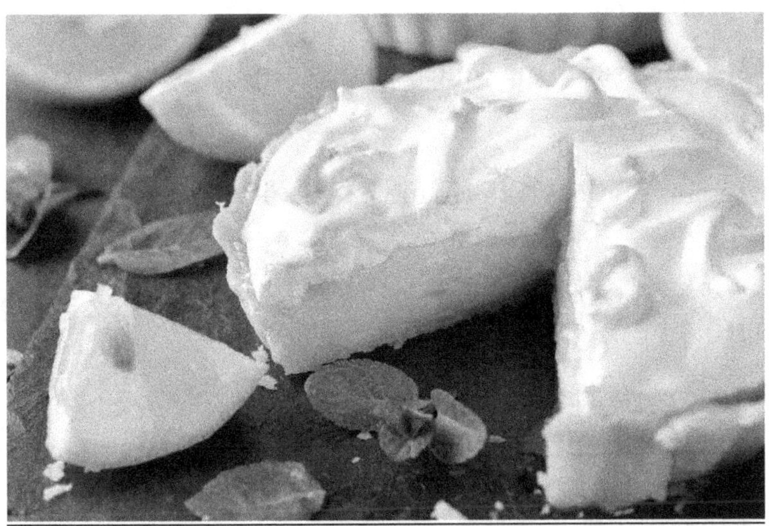

Ingredients:

<u>For the pie crust:</u>

1,8 oz (50 g) macadamia nuts

2,3 oz (65 g) butter

1 egg

0,88 oz (25 g) grated coconut

0,35 oz (10 g) coconut flour

2 pinches of stevia

2 pinches of baking soda

1 pinch of cinnamon

<u>For the lemon cream:</u>

2 small lemons

2 egg yolks, keep the whites for the meringue,

¼ tsp stevia

40 grams of room temperature butter, diced

The preparation:

For the pie crust:

- Take out the butter in advance to soften it.

- In a bowl: mix all the dry ingredients, add the egg, the butter and knead, you will get a shortbread dough

- Roll out the dough in the mold, press it well. (You can put the dough for a few hours in the fridge to harden it because it is quite crumbly)

Bake for about 15 minutes in the oven at 356 ° F (180 ° C).

For the lemon cream:

- Beat the egg yolks. Gradually add the lemon juice while stirring

- Put everything back on low heat and let thicken while stirring. When the mixture becomes very

creamy, remove from heat, add the pieces of butter
and mix powerfully

-    Let cool, then pour over the pie crust & you're
     done!

FATBOMBS WITH SEAWEED TARTARE

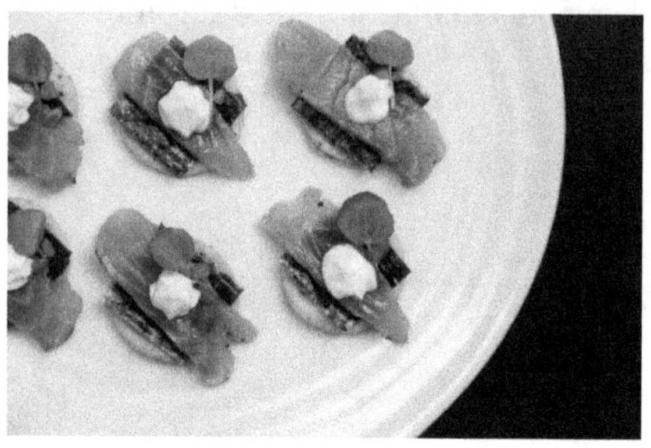

Ingredients:

1,8 oz (50 g) cocoa butter

1,2 oz (35) g ghee

0,5 oz (15 g) coconut oil

0,5 oz (15 g) coconut flour

1 tsp natural or lemon seaweed tartare

A little salt

A little powdered pepper

The preparation:

- Melt the cocoa butter, add the ghee and coconut oil. Add the rest of the ingredients and at the end the seaweed tartare → Mix

- distribute them in mini-molds. Let cool and put in
  the fridge to harden them

KETO COOKIES

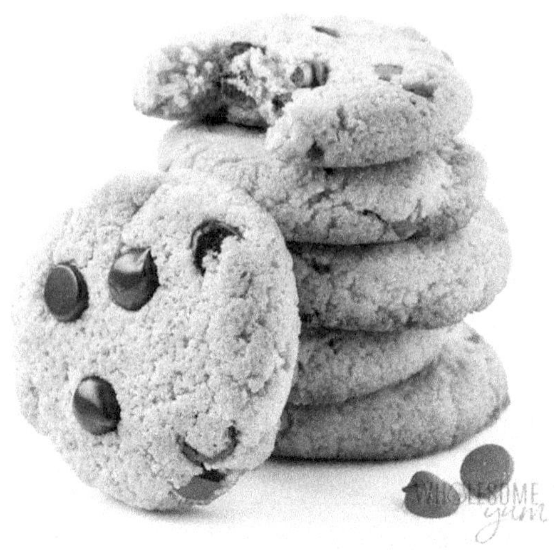

Ingredients:

3,5 oz (100 g) macadamia nuts

3,5 oz (100 g) butter

2 eggs

1,8 oz (50 g) grated coconut

0,7 oz (20 g) coconut flour

1/4 tsp stevia be very careful with stevia powder because it sugar a lot,

1/4 tsp baking soda

1 pinch of cinnamon

The preparation:

- Take out the butter in advance to soften it

- Crush the macadamia nuts to powder, the more you crush, the less crunchy they will be, so it's to your liking

- In a bowl: mix all the dry ingredients, add the butter and knead, you will get a shortcrust pastry

    o At this point, if you want shortbread, put the dough in cookie cutters, or make small shapes on baking paper. Put in the oven at 356 ° F (180 ° C) for about 15 minutes

- If you want soft cookies, add the two eggs, mix well and proceed as above.

AVOCADO OIL MAYONNAISE

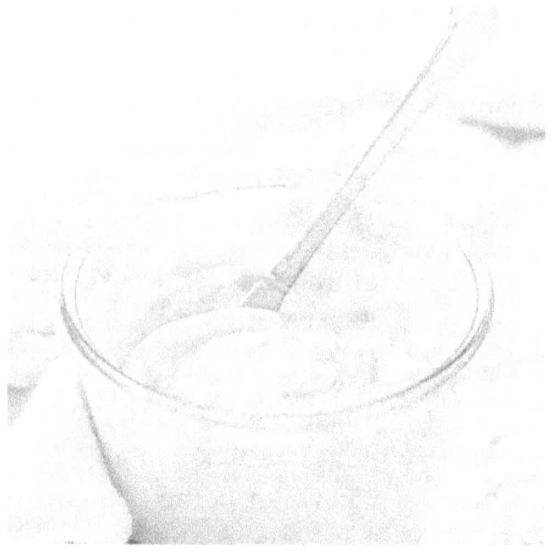

Ingredients:

1 egg

0,08 gal (300 ml) avocado oil

salt

1 tsp apple cider vinegar or lemon

The preparation:

- Break the egg in a bowl, add salt, 0,05 oz (200 ml) of oil & Mix until thickened

- Add the vinegar and the rest of the oil & mix

Mayonnaise can be stored for several days in the fridge.

LEMON CURD

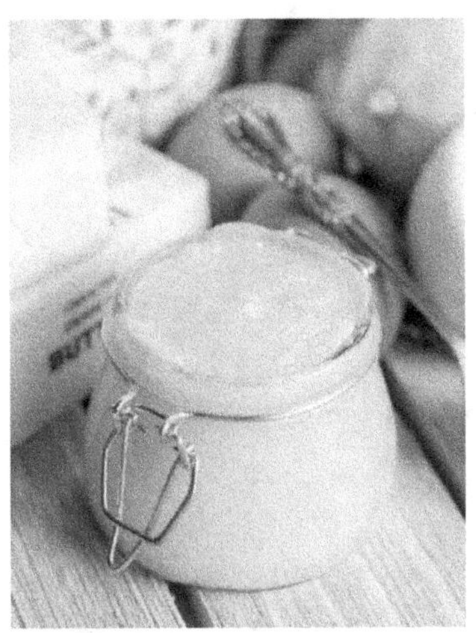

Ingredients:

1/2 avocado

1/3 glass of lemon curd

Some drops of stevia

0,013 gal (5 cl) of whole liquid cream

½ tsp of vanilla extract (optional)

The preparation:

- Mix the 1/2 avocado with a few drops of stevia (flavored with mint for me :)

- Whip the cream with a few drops of stevia and ½ tsp of vanilla extract in a bowl → add the lemon curd

-   Mix the liquid avocado with the whipped cream

46

Make your dessert by alternating the color as you wish. Either the avocado first, or the lemon curd. Keep cool until ready to serve

PUMPKIN CUPCAKES

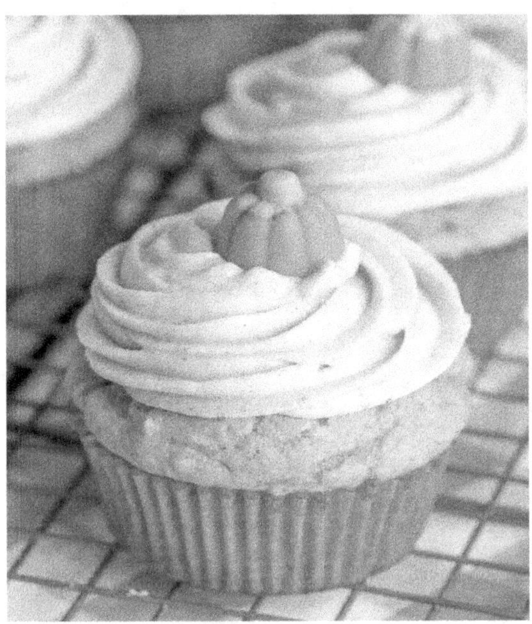

Ingredients:

<u>For cupcakes:</u>

7,1 oz (200 g) pumpkin puree (or a pumpkin)

4 eggs

1,1 oz (30 g) coconut flour

¼ tsp stevia powder

3,5 oz (100 g) butter

1 tsp baking soda

1 tsp spice for speculoos

1 tsp cinnamon powder

<u>For the coconut whipped cream:</u>

0,066 gal (250 ml) coconut cream

¼ tsp stevia

½ tsp of vanilla extract

The preparation:

For the cream:

- The day before, put the coconut cream in the fridge

- Pour the cream into the bowl, add the stevia and vanilla extract, whip everything until you get a whipped cream.

For the cupcake:

- Preheat the oven to 356 ° F (180 ° C)

- With a pumpkin (optional)
  - Prepare the pumpkin
    - Peel, remove the seeds, cut into cubes
  - Cook the pumpkin cubes in a pot of boiling water for about 20 minutes
  - Drain and mash them → pumpkin puree

- Mix the eggs and the butter → add the pumpkin puree, the spices, the stevia, the bicarbonate & mix again

-    Add the coconut flour & and mix one last time

-    Pour into cupcake molds or small muffins and bake
     for about 20 minutes. Prick with the blade of a knife
     to check the doneness.

You just have to decorate the cupcakes now.

KETOGENIC MAKIS

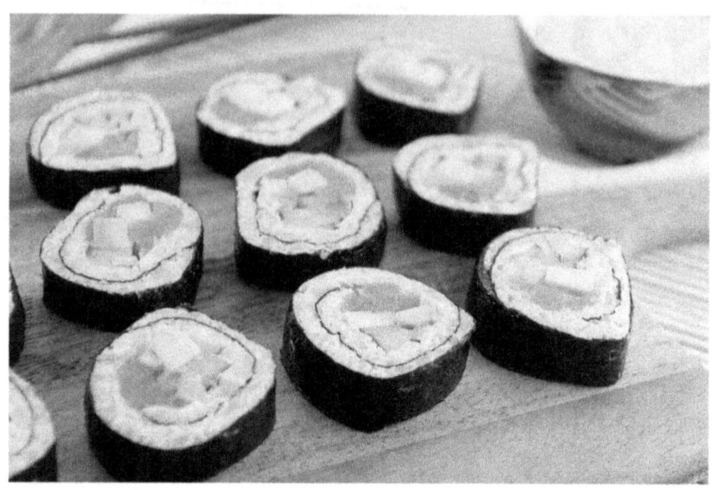

Ingredients:

2 Nori leaves

6 smoked salmon strips , about 1,4 oz (40 g)

6 cucumber strips about 0,35 oz (10g)

4,6 oz (130 g) cauliflower, coarsely mixed

The preparation:

- Spread the nori sheet on a work surface. With wet hands, put half the cauliflower on the end (about 1/4) of the leaf

- Put 3 salmon sticks on it, then 3 cucumbers

-    Roll up. Reserve in a cling film. Do the same for the second.

-    Put a few minutes in the fridge before cutting each roll into 6 using a wet knife

BACON DUMPLINGS

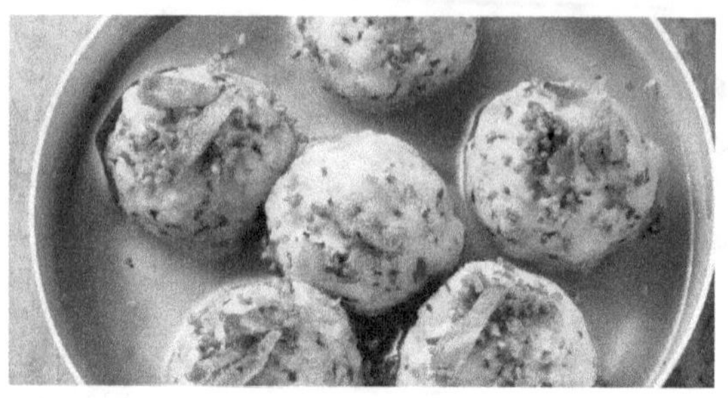

Ingredients:

14,1 oz (400 g) sausage meat

2 to 3 trays of 2,6 oz (75g) pancetta or bacon

12 dice of cheddar cheese (optional)

The preparation:

- Preheat the oven to 356 ° F (180 ° C)

- Make 10 to 12 small squares with the sausage meat on a baking sheet or baking mat

- Place a dice of cheddar on each square, form the balls. Surround each ball with pancetta (I put 4 on one ball)

- Bake for 20 to 25 minutes (the bacon should be nicely browned).

- Eat hot with or without sauce (mayonnaise, ketchup, etc.)

AVOCADO ICE CREAM

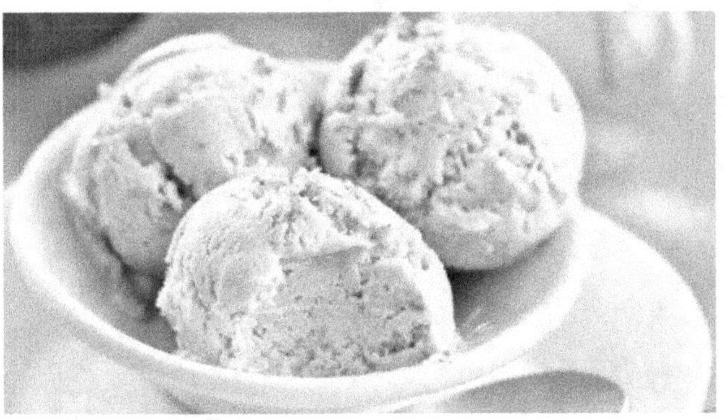

Ingredients:

1/2 avocado

2 jars of coconut yogurt

lime zest or mint flavor

a little stevia or other sweetener

The preparation:

- Mix the half avocado → pour the yogurts, the stevia and the lime zest or mint flavor & mix

  (it is difficult to put the right amount of stevia in a preparation, so it is better to put it little by little and add more rather than putting too much, then do not hesitate to taste your preparation)

- Put it in the fridge until it is frozen. This can take a couple of hours

BLACKBERRY CAKE, GLUTEN-FREE AND SUGAR-FREE

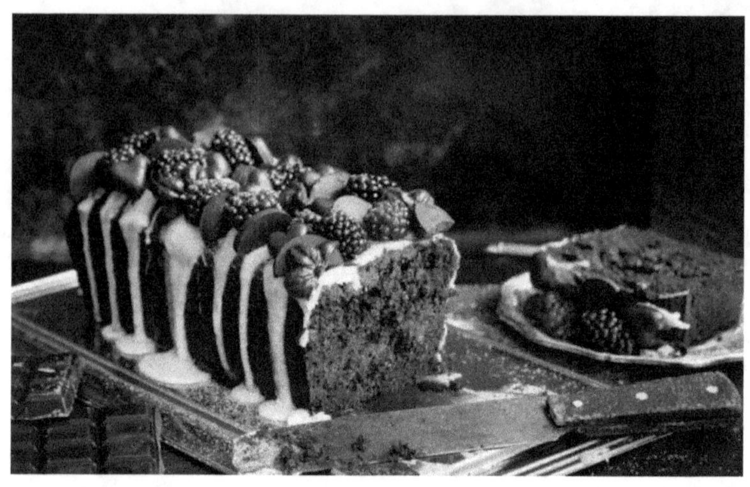

Ingredients:

3,5 oz (100 g) butter

3 eggs

1,2 oz (35 g) almond flour

0,7 oz (21 g) coconut flour

2,6 oz (75 g) xylitol

1,8 oz (50 g) or more blackberries

1 tsp baking soda

1 tsp lemon juice

lemon zest

The preparation:

- Put the previously melted butter in a bowl, add the xylitol and mix. Add the flours and baking soda & mix

- Add the whole eggs & mix

- Finally, add the lemon juice, lemon zest, the blackberries and mix one last time

- Pour into a small mold (about 16 cm in diameter). Bake in the preheated oven at 356 ° F (180 ° C) for about 30 minutes

SMOKED TROUT AND COCONUT MILK BROCCOLI

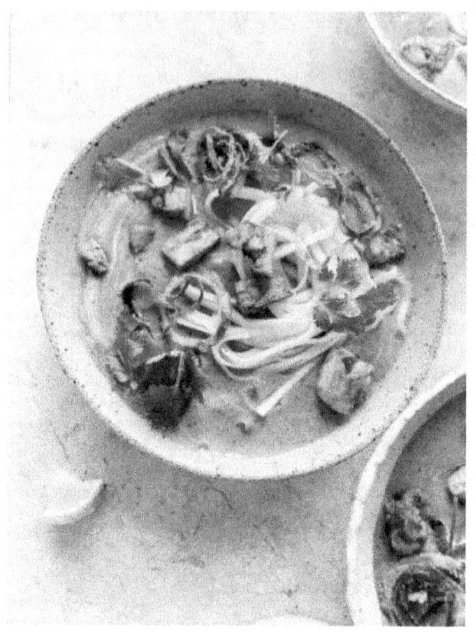

Ingredients:

8,8 oz (250 g) smoked trout or salmon or other fish fillet

3 eggs

7,1 oz (200 ml) coconut cream

1 bunch of broccoli

1 or 2 handful of spinach

2 tsp ghee or butter

2 tsp ginger paste

1 tsp coconut flour

1 tbs or more grated Parmesan cheese as desired

2 onions

salt

The preparation:

- Cut the broccoli and onions (in slices) and set aside

- Heat the ghee or the butter in a frying pan. Add the sliced onions, the ginger paste (or spice you want), mix well and add the broccoli

- Pour a little water and cook for a few minutes

- Then add the spinach leaves and the fish (in the same pan). Cook for another couple of minutes, turning from time to time until there is no more water.

- Mix the eggs with the cream and coconut flour in a bowl

- Pour everything from the bowl over the fish-broccoli mixture off the heat, add some salt

- Put in a gratin dish, sprinkle with Parmesan, and bake at 356 ° F (180 ° C) for about 20 minutes

FLOURLESS CHOCOLATE CAKE

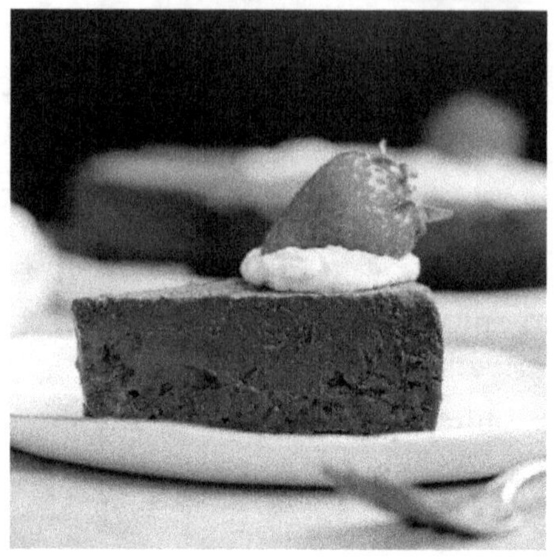

Ingredients:

Chocolate cake:

3,5 oz (100 g) of 100% Dark Chocolate

3,0 oz (85 g) Butter

0,2 oz (6 g) cocoa powder without sugar

2,5 oz (70 g) erythritol

6 eggs

Salt (optional)

Chocolate ream:

4,6 oz (130 g) dark chocolate 100%

13,2 oz (375 g) whole liquid cream

1 tsp of soluble coffee

25 g erythritol or 1/4 tsp stevia

The preparation:

<u>For the chocolate cake:</u>

- Melt the butter and chocolate, set aside

- Separate the egg yolks from the whites and whisk together the yolks with 0,7 oz (20 g) of erythritol and cocoa powder.

- Whisk the egg whites with the salt and the other 1,8 oz (50 g) of the erythritol in 3 different bowls

- Put 1/3 of the egg whites in the chocolate preparation and mix normally. Add the rest of the whites and mix gently.

- Line a baking plate with baking paper, pour the cake batter over it and bake at 356 ° F (180 ° C) (preheated oven) for 10 to 12 minutes. Take it out of the oven and let it cool

<u>Cream:</u>

- Melt the chocolate

- Add soluble coffee and erythritol/stevia to the liquid cream and whip it to whipped cream (Keep cream in the fridge before you start, makes the whipping easier)

- Mix the cream with the melted chocolate

Put the cream on the cake and you're done!

SOUFFLÉ WITH CELERIAC

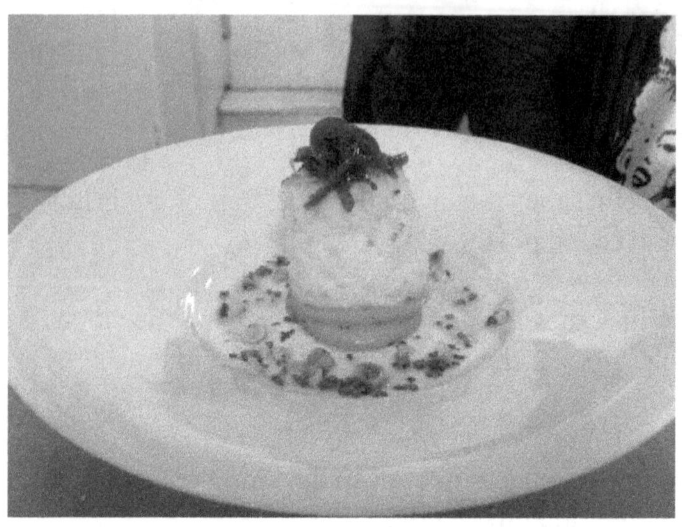

Ingredients:

10,6 oz (300 g) celeriac

3 tbs of fresh cream

2 eggs

0,7 oz (20 g) butter + butter for mussels

1,4 oz (40 g) of grated cheese

Pepper and salt

The preparation:

- Generously butter the ramekins (small bowls) and put them in the fridge

- Peel the celeriac, cut into cubes. Cook in a saucepan or steam and puree it

- Separate the egg yolks from the whites and mix them with the puree

- Add the butter, cream, grated cheese, salt and pepper & mix everything

- Whip the egg whites until stiff and pour them gently into the previous preparation. Divide among the ramekins and put in the oven preheated to 356 ° F (180 ° C) for about 30 minutes

Serve immediately.

COCONUT MILK SHRIMP

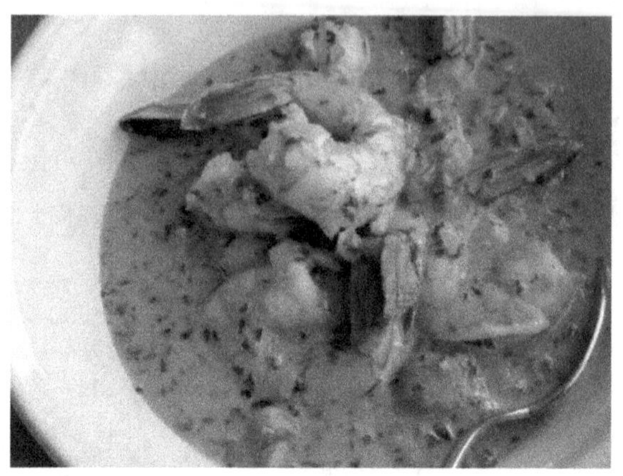

Ingredients:

0,066 gal (25cl) almond powder

0,066 gal (25 cl) coconut flour

2 tsp psyllium powder

2 tsp coconut oil

2 eggs

Roughly 5 tsp ice water

¼ tsp salt

For garnish:

2 leeks, about 9,5 oz (270 g)

8,8 oz (250 g) of trout or salmon fillet

5,3 oz (150 g) peeled shrimps

3 eggs

7,1 oz (200 ml) coconut cream

2 tsp ghee or butter

2 tsp curry paste

salt

The preparation:

- Combine all the dry ingredients in a bowl: almond powder, coconut flour, psyllium powder and salt

- Beat the 2 eggs in a small bowl and leave them aside

- Add 2 tsp of coconut oil to the dry ingredients and mix, you should have a sandy consistency. Add the eggs and mix well again.

- Pour in ice water until you reach a consistency where you can work with the dough (pour carefully)

- Knead well until you can form a ball, let stand 5 minutes

- Roll out the dough by flattening well to get a fairly fine bottom

- You can spread it between two baking sheets and transfer it delicately to the oven. Precook the dough for 12 to 15 minutes at 356 ° F (180 ° C)

For garnish:

While your dough is in the oven:

- cut and wash the white leeks, cut into pieces (not too small but not too large either)

- put the white leeks and cook for 1 to 2 minutes in some water. Then add the fish and shrimp, the curry paste and salt. Cook until the water is gone.

- In a bowl: beat the eggs with the coconut milk and mix

- Heat the ghee/butter in an oven dish, take your dough out of the oven and put it in the oven dish, add the filling with the fish to the fish on the dough and pour the egg and coconut milk mixture over it. Re-bake for 20 to 30 minutes at 356 ° F (180 ° C) until the top is golden.

Enjoy.

FATBOMB CHOCOLATES

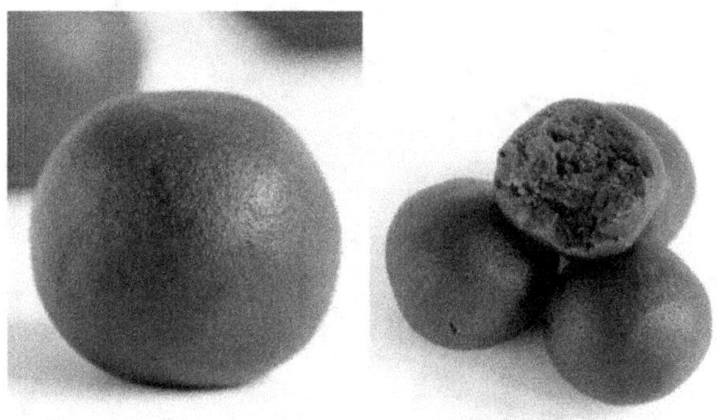

Ingredients:

2,5 oz (70 g) 100% chocolate

2,5 oz (70 g) cocoa butter

1 tbs coconut butter (about 30 g)

15 to 20 crushed macadamia nuts

The preparation:

- Coarsely crush the macadamia nuts (I do this with a knife)

- Melt the chocolate and cocoa butter together. Add the coconut butter and macadamia nuts & mix

- Pour into the mold, let cool and put the fridge to harden them. Easy, right? Enjoy!

CASTELLA CAKE

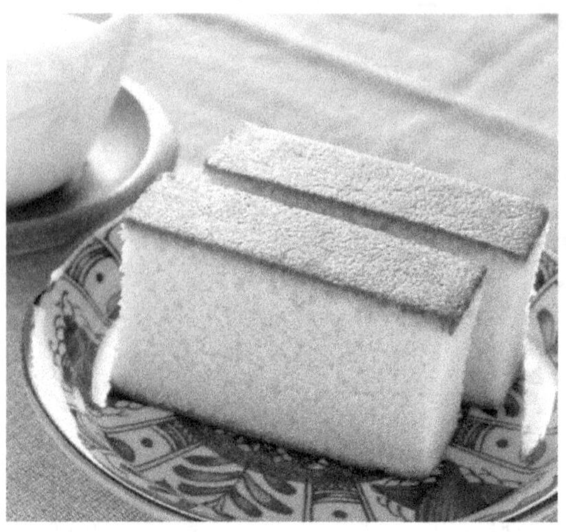

Ingredients:

6 eggs

3,5 oz (100 g) of butter

3,5 oz (100 g) of liquid cream

2,1 oz (60 g) of erythritol

1 tsp coffee vanilla extract

2,1 oz (60 g) coconut flour

The preparation:

- Separate the egg whites from the yolks

- Melt the butter with the cream (in the microwave or bain-marie), add the coconut flour & mix

- Add the egg yolks one by one, mixing well each
  time.

- Add the vanilla extract and whip the egg whites
  until stiff, gradually adding the sweetener. The
  whites do not have to be very firm

- Put 2 to 3 large spoons of egg whites in the egg yolk
  mixture and mix everything well. Then pour this
  mixture into the remaining egg whites and mix
  gently

- Pour everything into a high-edge mold covered with
  parchment paper (if you don't have a high-edge
  mold, make the parchment paper a few inches
  above the mold).

- Place the mold for 60 minutes in the oven preheated
  to 302 ° F (150 ° C)

FRID CHICKEN LIVERS

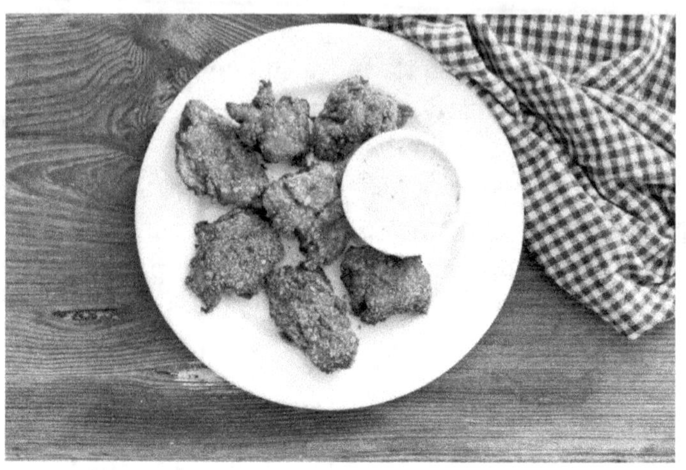

Ingredients:

14,1 oz (400 g) chicken livers

2 tsp of duck fat (or oil)

4 garlic cloves

0,7 oz (20 g) fresh ginger

1 tomato (optional)

1 shallot

1 tsp sweet paprika

1 tsp green pepper

The preparation:

- Grate peel and grate the ginger and garlic cloves, wring to take the juice.

- Season the chicken livers and marinate for 15 minutes or more

- Meanwhile cut the shallot and the tomato.

- When your casserole is on "hot": use the duck fat, brown the shallot, add the paprika & mix.

- Then add the chicken livers and mix for a few moments. Add the tomato, peppers & mix one last time

- Optional: Pour a little bit of water into the casserole dish, close it and use the pressure-cooking function on the "meat stew" function for 8 minutes
    o Cooked this way, the chicken livers will be tender.

MEAT WITH SPINACH

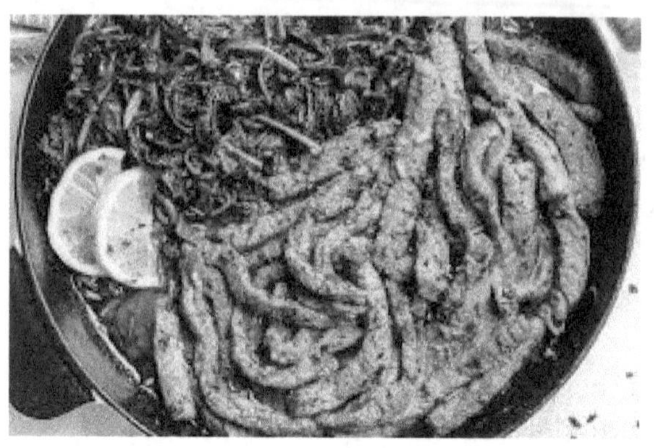

Ingredients:

17,6 oz (500 g) sausage or chicken meat

15 spinach leaves or 6 kale leaves

9 ham slices

9 cheese slices

1 egg

1 onion or 2 shallots

1 small bunch of fresh coriander

14 smoked port breast slices

Salt, pepper, ginger and/or chili

The preparation:

- Mix the meat (even if it is sausage meat) with the chopped onion, the egg, chopped cilantro, salt, pepper, ginger and/or chili

- Boil the spinach leaves in salted water, drain and set aside.

- Line a baking sheet with cling film. Spread the seasoned mixed meat & flatten to have a fairly thin layer

- Place the ham slices on the meat, then the cheeses and at the end the spinach leaves (or kale)

- Roll it all up with the plastic film (it's easier and it doesn't stick), shape the sausage well. Place the smoked breast slices on it and cover with aluminum foil.

- Bake at 356 ° F (180 ° C) for 30 minutes, take out the meat, remove the aluminum foil and return to the oven for another 30 minutes, this time at 392 ° F (200 ° C)

Take it out of the oven and serve hot & enjoy!

KETOGENIC CHOCOLATE LOG

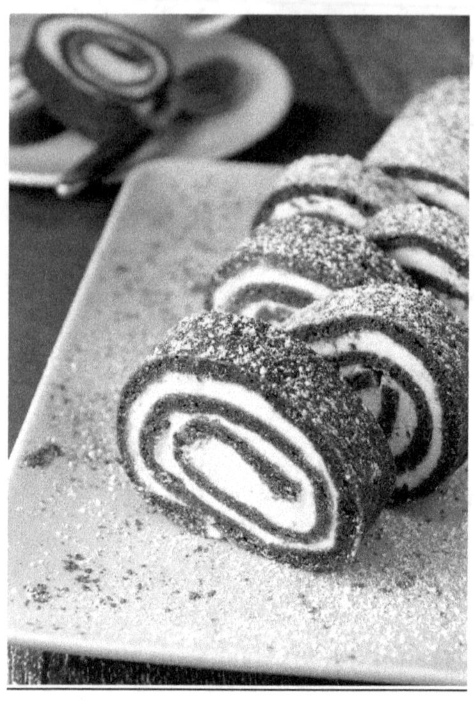

Ingredients:

<u>For the cookie:</u>

3,5 oz (100 g) butter

6 eggs

1,8 oz (50 g) 100% dark chocolate

2,5 oz (70 g) erythritol

1/4 tsp liquid stevia

1/2 tsp of food baking soda

1/4 tsp of gum mix (optional but makes the cake more flexible),

1/4 tsp apple cider vinegar (not essential if you use yeast),

1,1 oz (30 g) coconut flour.

For the chocolate cream:

2,5 oz (70 g) cocoa butter

2,5 oz (70 g) 100% chocolate

¼ tsp liquid stevia (or other sweetener)

0,066 gal (250 ml) liquid cream (adjust if too thick)

lime

The preparation:

The cookie:

- Melt the butter and chocolate, let cool

- Break 3 egg and separate the egg yolk form the white and put aside

- In a bowl: break 3 whole eggs and add the 3 egg yolks, mix them with the erythritol and liquid stevia until the mixture turns white

- Add the melted chocolate with the butter and the other ingredients except the coconut flour & mix

- Now add the coconut flour and add the whites that
  are beaten until stiff & mix

- Pour onto a baking sheet covered with parchment
  paper and bake for 10 to 15 minutes in the oven
  preheated to 356 ° F (180 ° C). As soon as it comes
  out of the oven, roll it with parchment paper and
  cover with a slightly damp cloth and let cool.

Chocolate cream:

The day before:

- melt the cocoa butter and chocolate

- Mix the cream with the sweetener and the squeezed
  lime

- Cover with cling film (the film should touch the
  cream), and put in the fridge

Finish:

Take out the chocolate cream and whip it up in whipped
cream. Unroll the cake, brush the inside of the chocolate
biscuit with the cream

Roll it again gently & enjoy!

SAVORY CAKE

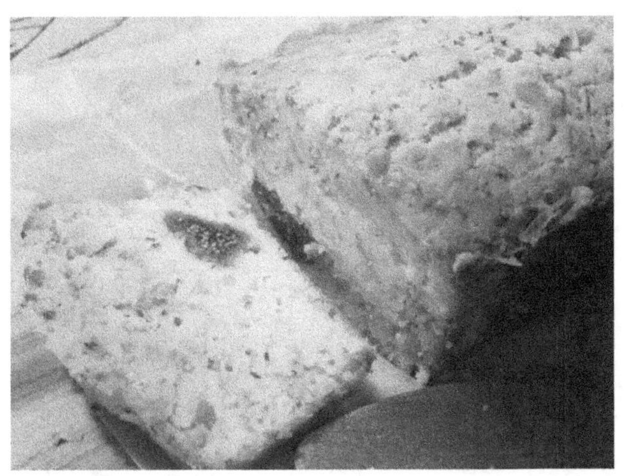

Ingredients:

4,4 oz (125 g) coconut flour

4,4 oz (125 g) butter

5 eggs

3,5 oz (100 g) milk kefir

1/4 tsp salt

1/4 tsp baking food

1/2 of optional gum mix

1/2 tsp ground ginger

The preparation:

- Melt the butter

- In a bowl: break the eggs and beat them until the mixture turns white. Add the butter and kefir & mix

- Add all the other ingredients and mix again

- Pour everything into a buttered pan and put in the preheated oven at 356 ° F (180 ° C) for about 30 minutes

Let cool & enjoy!

MID-KETO KETOGENIC

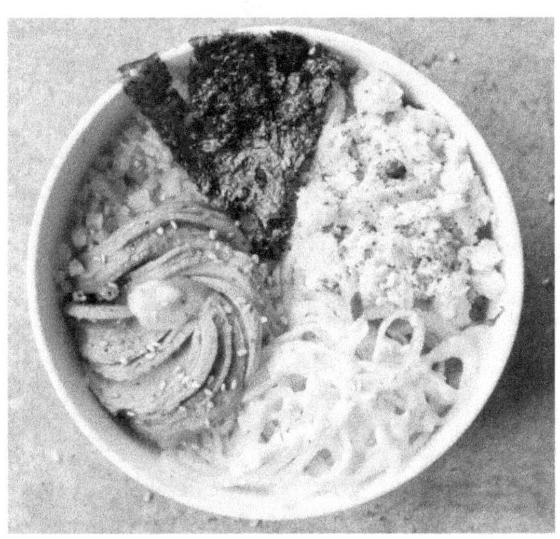

Ingredients:

A box of Shirataki noodles

1,4 oz (40 g) butter + 0,35 oz (10 g) butter for the omelet

2,5 oz (70 g) roast pork chop or other meats

1 egg

5,3 oz (150 g) of Chinese cabbage or other vegetables

salt and pepper

some coriander leaves or parsley

The preparation:

- Prepare the shirataki as directed on the box and set aside

-   Make an omelet with the egg, cut into small pieces
    and set aside

-   Chop the Chinese cabbage, coriander leaves, and
    meat

-   In a pan with the 1,4 oz (40 g) melted butter, add
    the Chinese cabbage & cook for a few minutes

-   Add the shirataki, salt and pepper, add the meat
    while mixing each time → add the coriander leaves
    & mix one last time

-   Put everything in a serving dish and decorate with
    the omelet.

There you go, it's ready, all you have to do is serve.

ZUCCHINI-FETA MUFFINS

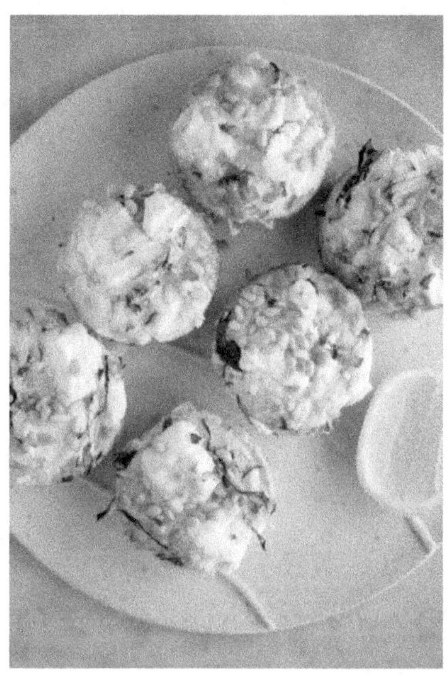

Ingredients:

7,1 oz (200 g) zucchini

1,8 oz (50 g) coconut flour

1,8 oz (50 g) butter

3 eggs

1,1 oz (30 g) feta cheese

1 tsp baking soda or ½ sachet baking powder

Salt

Aromatic herbs or other spices

Chili (optional)

The preparation:

- Melt the butter and let cool

- Grate the zucchini with the cheese grater

- In a bowl: the melted butter, eggs, coconut flour, baking soda, salt and chili & mix everything

- Add the grated zucchini and the diced feta cheese & mix one last time

- Put in the preheated oven at 356 ° F (180 ° C) for about 20 minutes

RASPBERRY ONION CONFIT

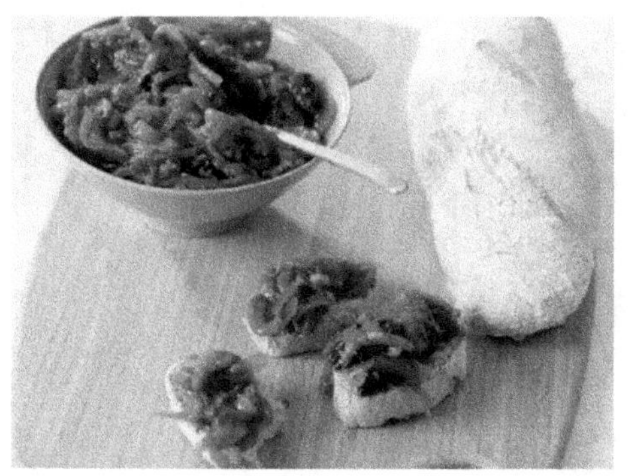

Ingredients:

0,7 oz (20 g) butter

0,7 oz (20 g) raspberry

salt

1 tsp apple cider vinegar

1,8 oz (50 g) onions

The preparation:

- Wash, peel and cut the onions

- Heat the butter in a pan → add the onions, salt & cook with some water

- When the onions are translucent add the raspberries and allow to reduce, stirring occasionally

- Remove from the heat when there is no more liquid

GINGERBREAD WITHOUT HONEY

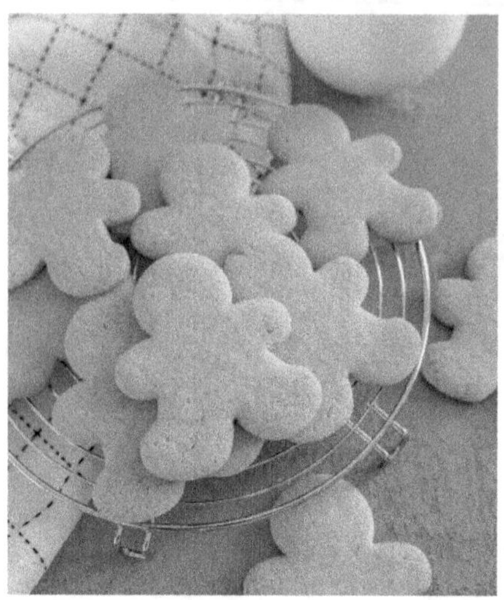

Ingredients:

2,1 oz (60 g) butter

7,1 oz (200 g) coconut milk

0,7 (20 g) erythritol or another sweetener

4 eggs

3,0 oz (85 g) coconut flour

1/4 tsp stevia powder

2 tsp gingerbread spices

1 tsp baking powder (yeast or bicarbonate)

The preparation:

- Melt the butter with erythritol over normal heat in a saucepan, stir until the mixture turns brown → remove from the heat and pour the coconut milk

- Separate the egg whites from the yolks.

- In a bowl: whip the egg yolks with the stevia powder → add the caramel (butter, erythritol, coconut milk) & continue to whip to mix well

- Add the coconut flour, baking powder and spices & mix → add the beaten egg whites & mix

- Pour everything into a buttered baking plate and press it flat

- Put in the preheated oven at 356 ° F (180 ° C) for about 15 to 20 minutes

- Use cookie molds to create the cookies of your dreams!

COCONUT AND MACADAMIA BITES

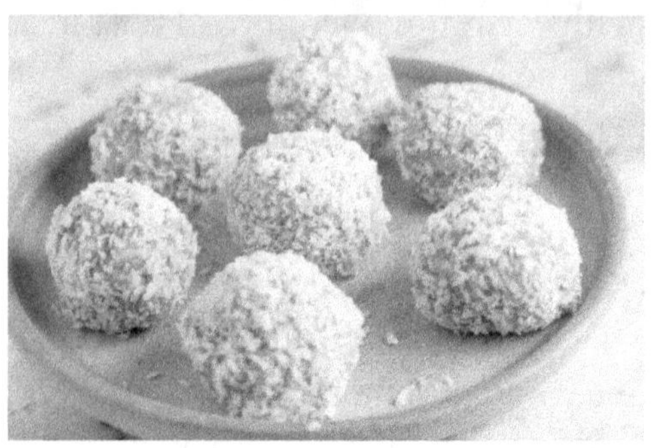

Ingredients:

0,16 gal (600 ml) of 80% coconut milk

¼ tsp stevia (optional)

5,3 oz (150 ml) concentrated coconut milk

4,4 oz (125 g) grated coconut

Dumpling dough for 12 to 14 dumplings

12 to 14 macadamia nuts

The preparation:

- Reduce the coconut milk in a saucepan over low heat. Stir from time to time until it is reduced to half → It will change a little color, it's normal. If you let it reduce even more, it will get fatter. Remove from the heat and add the stevia & mix

- Mix the grated coconut with the sweetened condensed milk you made in the step above → put in a bowl or on a plate

- Shape 14 dumplings, insert a macadamia nut in each dumpling, roll them in the coconut mix the bowl or plate

Keep cool if you don't eat them right away.

FILLET OF BEEF, PEANUT-SESAME PESTO

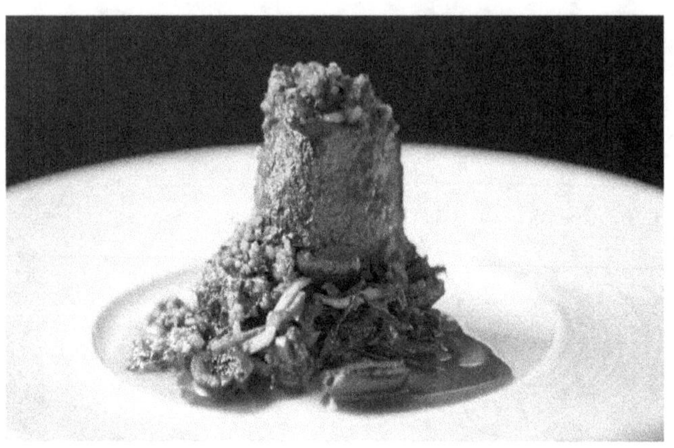

Ingredients:

28,2 oz (800 g) beef tenderloin

3,5 oz (100 g) roasted peanuts

2,8 oz (80 g) sesame

4 garlic cloves

1 onion with the stem

1 piece of ginger

1 carrot

1 celery stalk

1 bunch of coriander

6 tbs chili ketchup

olive oil

Pepper & salt

The preparation:

- Preheat the oven to 464 ° F (240 ° C)

- Mix the peanuts, sesame, garlic, onion, ginger, sliced carrot, celery, cilantro, salt, pepper until you have a thin mince.

- Coat the fillet with ketchup, roll it in the mince and sprinkle with a drizzle of olive oil and bake in the oven: 15 minutes; very rare, 20 minutes; rare, 25 minutes less rare… let stand 5 minutes before putting it cut.

SALMON-AVOCADO RILLETTES

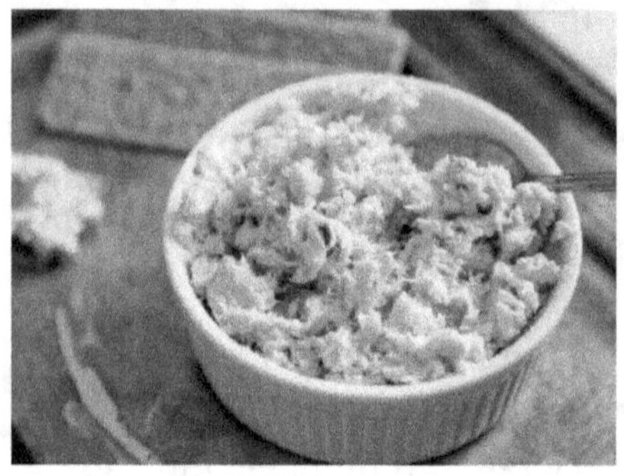

Ingredients:

14,1 oz (400 g) fresh salmon flesh

0,13 gal (50 cl) shellfish broth

2 avocados

1 shallot

juice of 1/2 lemon

2 tbs of olive oil

0,35 oz (10 g) butter

1 kiwi

1 tonka bean

0,026 gal (10 cl) white wine

few drops tabasco

0,026 gal (10 cl) whipping cream

0,026 gal (10 cl) heavy cream

few sprigs chickweed

The preparation:

- Simmer the shellfish broth and add the salmon for 15 minutes without boiling, but heating

- Remove from heat, drain the fish with a slotted spoon → let it cool before crumbling it with a fork

- Peel and chop the shallot. Mix it with the butter and olive oil → pour the wine. Leave to reduce for 5 minutes and put aside

- Peel and cut the kiwi into small dice.

- Mix the salmon with the shallot in the white wine, add the 2 creams and 1 pinch of grated tonka bean. Add the diced kiwi, salt & pepper

- Cover with cling film and set aside in the fridge for 2 hours

- Split the avocados in half, pit them and remove the skin, lemon the flesh lightly and cut it into 1 cm cubes. Sprinkle with a few drops of Tabasco & mix gently so as not to crush the diced avocado

- Add delicately to the preparation of salmon, sprinkle with chickweed

Enjoy!

TUNA MARINATED IN SPICES

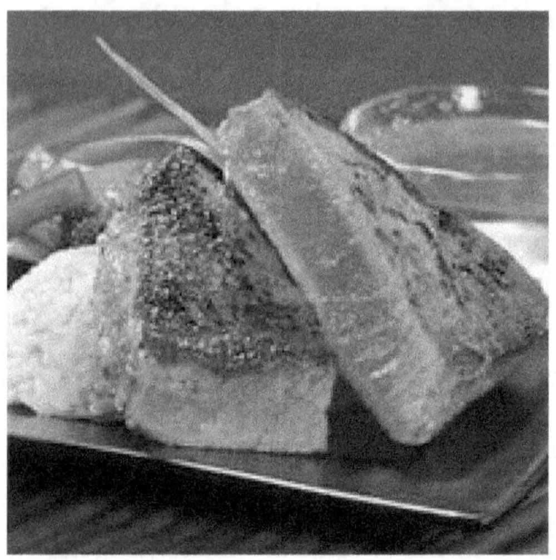

Ingredients:

14,1 oz (400 g) of tuna red line

1 lemon

1 tsp caraway/cumin seeds

2 tsp of salt

1 pinch of chili

1 small piece of ginger root

2 tsp of olive oil

The preparation:

- Grate the ginger → add: lemon juice, caraway/cumin seeds, salt, chili and olive oil & mix

- Cut the tuna into slices (the finer it is, the more the tuna will be cooked; to your liking)

- Place the cooked tuna in a salad bowl, drizzle with marinade. Cover with film and let marinate overnight.

Serve the next day with a few sprigs of dill and possibly borage flowers

WILD PINK SALMON IN PARMESAN

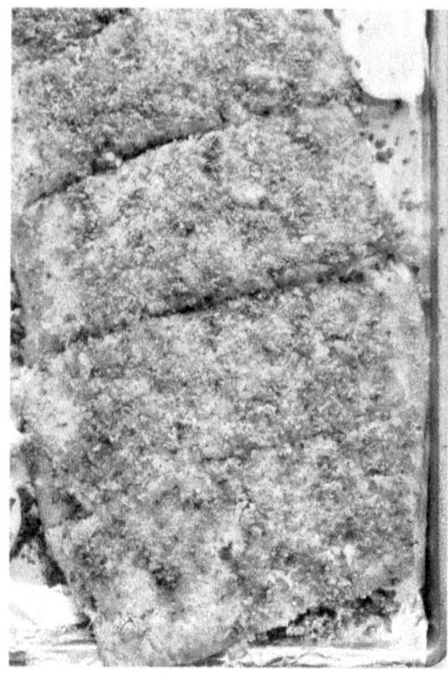

Ingredients:

4 North Pacific pink wild salmon fillets

strong Dijon mustard

1 tsp pepper

4 tsp of breadcrumbs

2 tsp very finely chopped parsley

1 tsp grated parmesan

1 large knob of sweet butter

7,1 oz (200 g) of egg

0,026 gal (10 cl) of cream liquid

1 small bunch of fresh savory

Salt

The preparation:

- Preheat the oven to 437 ° F (225 ° C)

- Season the salmon fillets with salt and pepper on all sides.

- Melt the butter in a pan and then brown the salmon fillets for a few minutes, turning them regularly

- Put salmon fillets in aluminium foil and cook for 4 to 5 minutes in the oven

- Meanwhile, prepare the breading in a bowl, mixing the breadcrumbs, finely chopped parsley, grated parmesan and 1 teaspoon pepper

- After 4 to 5 minutes, remove the salmon fillets from the oven. Do not turn off the oven, and keep it at 437 ° F (225 ° C)

- Arrange the salmon fillets on a work surface, allowing them to cool for a few moments and remove the foil

- Then coat each fillet of salmon with strong mustard with Dijon using a kitchen brush and cover them well with the breading mixture

- Put the salmon fillets on a dish again in aluminium foil and let them cook for another 4 to 5 minutes in the oven at 437 ° F (225 ° C)

-   In a small skillet, reduce the fresh cream mixed with
    the thinly sliced savory by half (over medium heat)
    & mix

-   Off the heat, briefly mix the cream and savory
    mixture with the Alaskan cod eggs

-   Place a few spoonsful of the vegetable cream and
    cod eggs in the center of each plate.

-   Place a salmon fillet over it, sprinkled with a pinch
    of salt, and serve immediately

LAMB CHOPS AND PISTACHIO PESTO

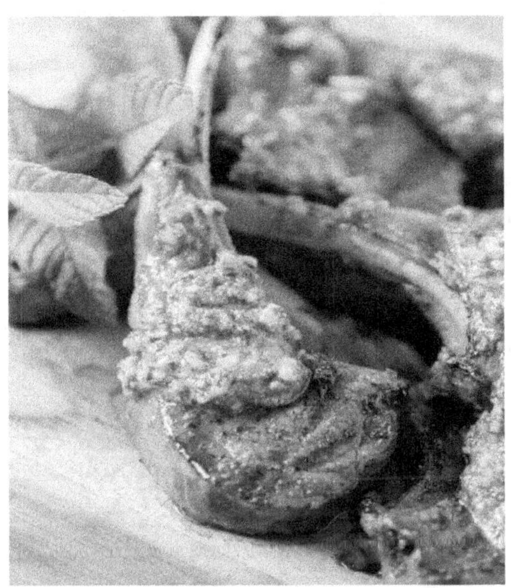

Ingredients:

12 lamb chops

1,8 oz (50 g) hulled pistachios

1 clove of garlic

1 bunch of basil

17,6 oz (500 g) small potatoes

1 bunch of new onions

salt

olive oil

freshly ground pepper

The preparation:

- Mix the pistachios, garlic, basil leaves with a little salt and pepper, adding a drizzle of olive oil to obtain a paste. Cover the chops

- Cook the potatoes and small onions (keep the stems) in a casserole dish with a drizzle of olive oil, about 30 minutes

- 10 minutes before the end of the cooking of the potatoes, salt with salt, pepper and add the finely chopped onion stalks

- Cook the chops in a non-stick pan for 3-4 minutes on each side and serve immediately

AROMATIC KETOGENIC ENERGY BALLS

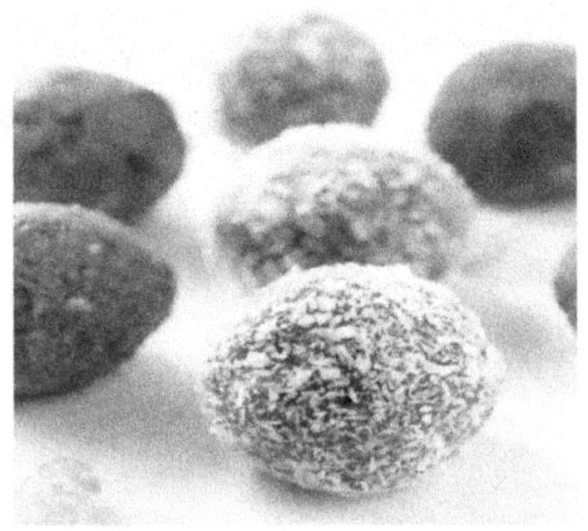

Ingredients:

7,9 oz (225 g) almond butter

0,06 gal (240 ml) coconut butter

3,4 oz (95 g) grated coconut

1 tsp organic vanilla extract

1 drop of cinnamon essential oil

Stevia (as needed, to taste)

The preparation:

- Soften the coconut butter (be careful not to melt)

- Mix all ingredients

- Form balls on a baking sheet

- Then store in the freezer

ALMOND POWDER BREAD

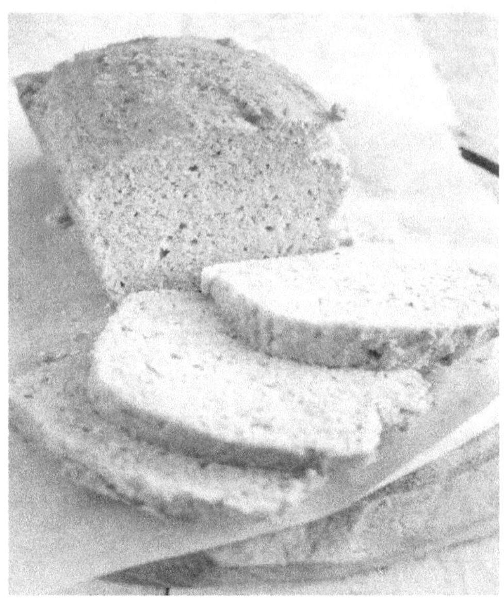

Ingredients:

2 egg whites (at room temperature)

2 eggs (at room temperature)

7,1 oz (200 g) almond flour

2,1 oz (60 g) melted butter

4 tsp psyllium / 2 tsp psyllium husk powder

1 1/2 tsp baking powder

1/2 tsp xanthan gum

pinch of salt

0,032 gal (120 ml) lukewarm water

The preparation:

- Preheat your oven to 356 ° F (180 ° C)

- Beat the 2 eggs and the 2 egg whites

- Add the other ingredients and mix them until a smooth paste is obtained. (Do not mix too much)

- Place in a cake mold covered with butter and put in the oven for about 45 minutes

COCONUT FLOURKETOGENIC BREAD

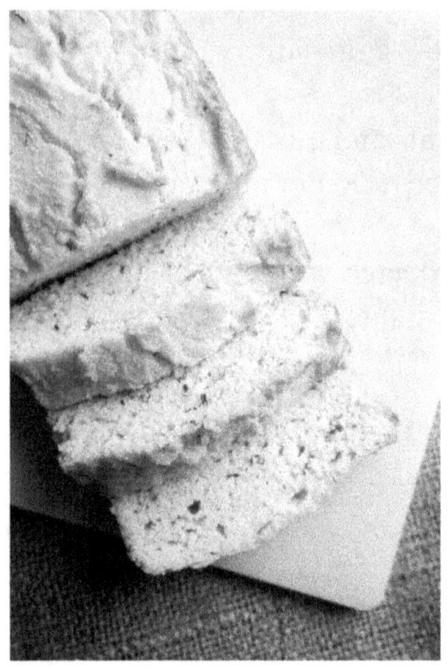

Ingredients:

3,5 oz (100g) of coconut flour

0,7 oz (20 g) of blond psyllium

2,1 oz (60 g) butter

2 eggs

¼ tsp cumin

¼ tsp garlic powder

½ tsp apple cider vinegar (optional)

½ tsp baking powder or yeast

17,6 oz (500 g) of hot water

The preparation:

- Preheat the oven to 356 ° F (180 ° C)

- Put all the dry ingredients in a bowl & mix → add the melted butter, the vinegar and the two eggs & mix again

- Then gradually pour in the hot water and mix until it forms a ball

- Put this mix in a cake mold and place it in the oven for about 1 hour

KETO SATAY CHICKEN

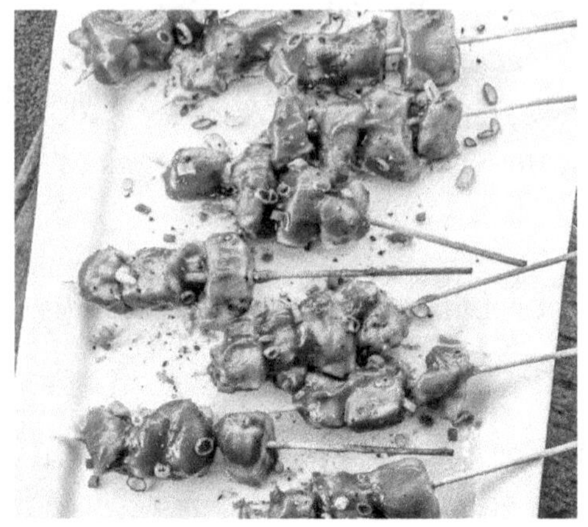

Ingredients:

1 1/2 tbs peanut oil

2 garlic cloves, crushed

1 tsp curry powder

1 tsp finely grated fresh ginger

2 (4,4 oz (125 g) each) chicken thigh fillets

1/4 red onion, finely chopped

1/2 small fresh red chili, deseeded, finely chopped

1 tsp peanut butter

0,02 gal (80 ml) coconut milk

1 tsp soy sauce

1 1/2 tsp chopped roasted salted peanuts

1/4 lime, juiced

1 large zucchini, trimmed

1/2 Lebanese cucumber, thinly sliced

4,4 oz (125g) cherry tomatoes, halved

The preparation:

-   Combine 1 tsp oil, 1 garlic clove, 1/2 tsp curry powder
    and the ginger in a shallow glass or ceramic dish → add
    the chicken and turn to coat

-   Cover and place in the fridge for at least one hour to
    marinate.

-   Heat the remaining oil in a small saucepan over medium
    heat → cook the onion, stirring, for 3 minutes or until
    softened → add the chili and the remaining garlic and
    curry powder and cook, stirring, for 1 minute or until
    aromatic.

-   Now add the peanut butter, coconut milk and soy sauce.
    Simmer, while stirring, for 2-3 minutes or until
    thickened slightly

-   Reserve 1 tsp chopped peanuts for serving

-   Stir the remaining peanuts and the lime juice into the
    sauce. Set aside, covered to keep warm.

-   Meanwhile, use a spiralizer to cut the zucchini into long
    noodles or cut the zucchini lengthwise with a vegetable
    peeler then cut into long strips

-   Heat a chargrill pan or barbecue over medium-high heat.
    Cook the chicken for 3-4 minutes each side or until
    lightly charred and cooked through. Transfer to a plate

and set aside to rest for 5 minutes before slicing the
chicken thickly

- Divide the zucchini 'noodles' among bowls → place the
  chicken on the zucchini → place the cucumber and
  tomatoes on the chicken → then drizzle with the warm
  satay sauce

KETO FRAPPUCCINO SLICE

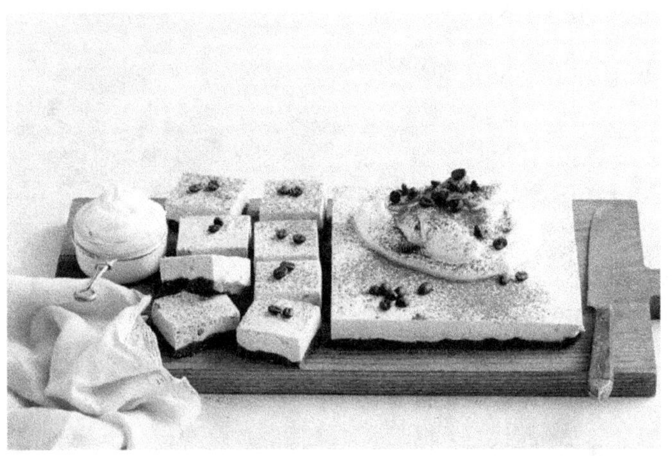

Ingredients:

<u>Cream</u>

2 tsp boiling water

2 1/2 tsp gelatin powder

8,8 oz (250 g) cream cheese, at room temperature, chopped

2 tsp powdered stevia

0,02 gal (80 ml) strong espresso coffee, cooled

1 tsp vanilla extract

0,079 gal (300 ml) thickened cream, whipped + a bit extra, whipped, to serve

Coffee beans, to serve (optional)

Cacao powder, to dust

<u>Base</u>

3,5 oz (100 g) pecans

4,6 oz (130 g) almond meal

1 tsp cacao powder

1 tsp powdered stevia

1 egg

2 tsp unsalted butter, melted

The preparation:

- Preheat oven to 356°F/320°F (180°C/160°C) fan forced. Line a 6,30 x 10,24 inch (16 x 26 cm) slice pan with baking paper, allowing the paper to overhang the 2 long sides

- To make the base, place the pecans in a food processor and process until finely ground

- Add the almond meal, cacao and stevia & mix to combine → add the egg and butter. Process until mixture comes together

- Transfer to prepared pan. Evenly press mixture firmly into the base. Bake for 10 minutes or until light golden. Set aside to cool

- Place the boiling water in a small heatproof bowl. Sprinkle over the gelatin and whisk until gelatin dissolves

-   Use electric beaters to beat the cream cheese, stevia, cooled coffee and vanilla in a large bowl until smooth

-   Now add the gelatin & mix until well combined. Fold in the whipped cream. Pour the mixture over the cooled base and use a spatula to smooth the surface

-   Cover and place in the fridge for 4 hours or until set.

-   Top with extra whipped cream and coffee beans, if using. Serve dusted with cacao

KETO LEMON MUG CAKE

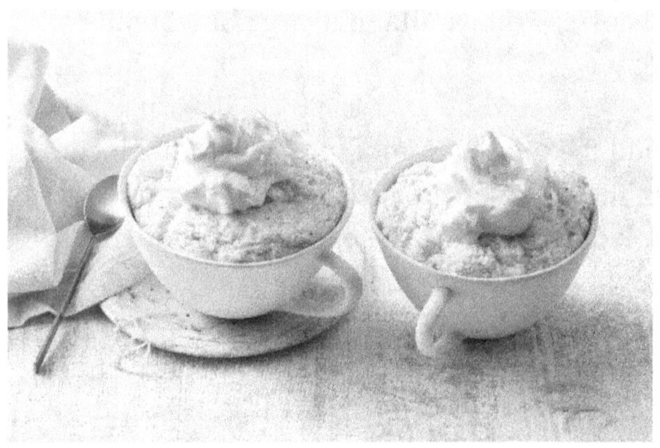

Ingredients:

0,7 oz (20 g) butter, melted, cooled

1 egg

1 tsp finely grated lemon rind, plus extra zested, to serve (optional)

0,88 oz (25 g) coconut flour

1 tsp ground almonds

2 tsp xylitol

1/2 tsp baking powder

2 tsp almond milk

1 tsp fresh lemon juice

Mascarpone, to serve

The preparation:

-   Whisk together the butter, egg and lemon rind in a small mixing bowl until combined → add the flour, almond, xylitol, baking powder, milk and juice & mix

-   Transfer mixture to a 0,066 gal (250 ml) heatproof mug or cup and smooth the surface. Microwave on HIGH for 2 minutes. Set aside for 30 seconds. Top with a dollop of mascarpone and extra lemon zest, if using, to serve.

KETO GARLIC BREAD

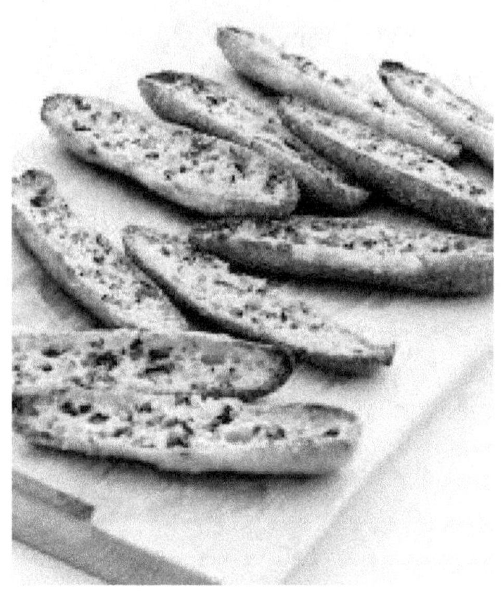

Ingredients:

0,25 oz (7 g) sachet instant dried yeast

1 tsp pouring cream

0,021 gal (80 ml) warm water

5,5 oz (155 g) almond meal

2 tsp syllium husk

1 tsp ground flaxseed

1 tsp baking powder

1/2 tsp table salt

3 eggs, lightly whisked

2 tsp olive oil

2 tsp apple cider vinegar

3 garlic cloves, finely chopped

2 tsp olive oil

3,5 oz (100 g) shredded mozzarella cheese

Chopped continental parsley, to serve

The preparation:

- Grease and line a square 7,87 inch (20cm) cake
  mold with baking paper

- Place the yeast, cream and water in a small bowl.
  Whisk to combine. Set aside for 10 minutes or until
  slightly frothy

- In a large bowl, whisk together the almond meal,
  psyllium husk, flaxseed, baking powder and salt →
  now make a well in the middle and add the yeast
  mixture, egg, olive oil and vinegar. Whisk well to
  combine

- Transfer to the mold and set aside for 1 hour or until
  the mix has risen slightly

- Preheat the oven to 392°F/356°F (200°C/180°C) fan
  forced. Bake the bread for 15 minutes

-   Drizzle with olive oil, sprinkle with garlic and scatter with cheese. Bake for a further 10 minutes or until cheese is bubbling

-   Sprinkle with parsley to serve

KETO TACO SHELLS

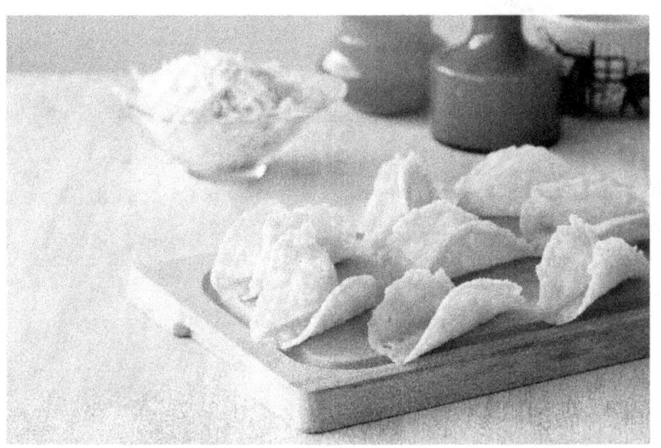

Ingredients:

2,1 oz (60 g) baby spinach leaves

2 eggs

1,4 oz (40g) almond meal

2 tsp psyllium husk

1/2 tsp salt

The preparation:

- Preheat oven to 356°F/320°F (180°C/160°C) fan forced. Line 2 baking trays with baking paper

- Place the spinach in a heatproof bowl. Pour over boiling water to cover. Set aside for 5 minutes to blanch → let it drain and squeeze out the extra liquid

- Transfer the spinach to the bowl of a food processor. Add the eggs, almond meal, psyllium husk and salt & Process until smooth

- Place one 1/4 of the mixture onto one of the prepared trays. Use a cranked spatula to spread to make a 5,91 inch (15 cm) circle

- Repeat with the remaining mixture to make 4 circles. Bake for 10 minutes

- Use a spatula to transfer the circles between the gaps of an upturned non-stick muffin pan to create a taco shape

- Set aside to cool slightly. Bake for a further 10 minutes to dry out

Fill with your favorite taco ingredients.

KETO STRAWBERRY CHEESECAKE BALLS

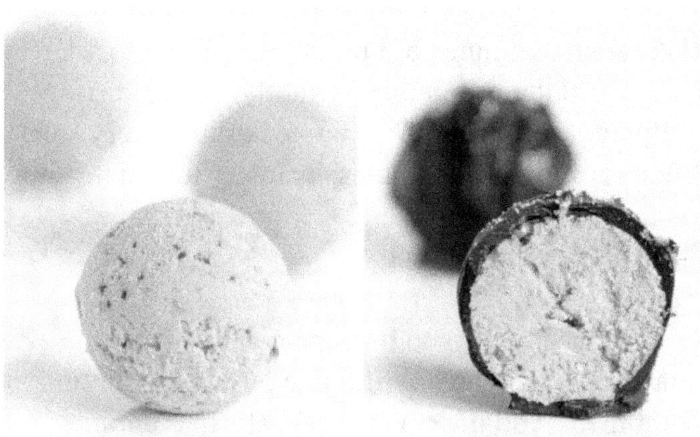

Ingredients:

12,3 oz (350 g) strawberries

8,8 oz (250 g) cream cheese, at room temperature, chopped

1 tsp xylitol

1,2 oz (35 g) desiccated coconut, plus 1 tsp extra

1,6 oz (45 g) pecans, finely chopped

The preparation:

- Preheat oven to 356°F/320°F (180°C/160°C) fan forced. Line a baking tray with baking paper

- Reserve 2 medium strawberries. Cut the remaining strawberries into quarters (or sixths if large) and place on the prepared tray

- Bake for 10 minutes or until starting to soften. Use a fork to flatten each piece slightly. Bake, stirring halfway, for a further 20 minutes or until very soft. Bake for a final 10 minutes. Transfer to a plate and set aside to cool completely → now you have strawberry pulp

- Use electric beaters to beat the cream cheese, strawberry pulp and xylitol in a large bowl until combined. Add the coconut and stir to combine

- Cover and place in the fridge for 1 hour or until firm

- Line a baking tray with baking paper. Cut the reserved strawberries in half lengthways then cut each half into quarters

- Take a level tablespoonful of the chilled cheesecake mixture and press a piece of fresh strawberry into the centre → roll into a ball and place on the prepared tray

- Repeat with remaining mixture and strawberry pieces.

- Place the extra coconut in a dish and the chopped pecan in another dish. Roll half the balls in pecan

and the other half in coconut, pressing lightly to
coat

- Place in the fridge and chill until firm. Store in an
airtight container in the fridge for up to 2 days

KETO CREAMY CHICKEN AND CAULIFLOWER SALAD

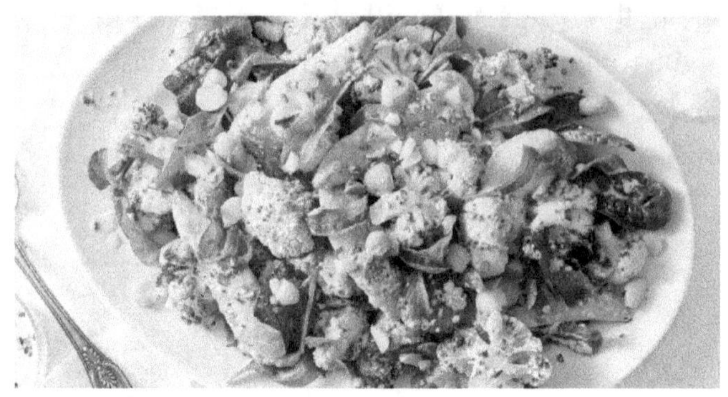

Ingredients:

17,6 oz (500 g) cauliflower, cut into florets

2 tsp olive oil

1 tsp Massel chicken style stock powder

0,021 gal (80 ml) Massel chicken-style stock

0,021 gal (80ml) pure cream

3 tsp wholegrain mustard

1 tsp chopped fresh chives, plus extra to serve

2 tsp lemon juice

14,1 oz (400 g) chicken tenderloins

3,5 oz (100 g) streaky bacon

3,5 oz (100 g) baby spinach

3,5 oz (100 g) rocket leaves

2,1 oz (60 g) roasted macadamia nuts, chopped

The preparation:

- Preheat oven to 392°F/356°F (200°C/180°C) fan forced. Line a baking tray with baking paper

- Place cauliflower on the prepared tray. Drizzle with 1 ½ tsp oil and sprinkle with the stock powder → bake for 25 minutes or until golden and tender

- Meanwhile, place stock and mustard in a small saucepan and bring to the boil over high heat → reduce heat and simmer for 2 minutes → add cream and simmer for a further 2-3 minutes or until sauce is reduced by half. Stir through chives and lemon juice, keep warm.

- Heat remaining oil in large non-stick frying pan over medium-high heat. Cook chicken and bacon for 3-4 minutes each side or until golden and crisp. Cut bacon into 1,18 inch (3 cm) pieces

- Arrange salad leaves, chicken, cauliflower and bacon on a serving platter. Drizzle with the cream sauce and sprinkle with macadamia nuts and remaining chives.

KETO SWEDISH MEATBALLS

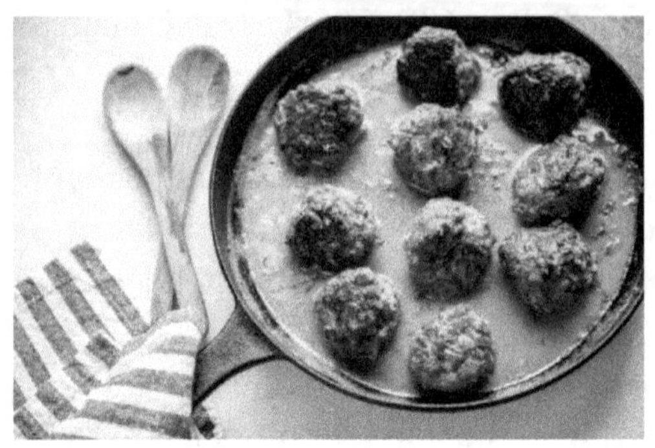

Ingredients:

17,6 oz (500 g) beef mince

1 egg

4 green shallots, thinly sliced

1/4 tbs finely chopped fresh continental parsley

1 garlic clove, crushed

1 tsp allspice

1/4 tsp ground nutmeg

2 tsp extra virgin olive oil

0,021 gal (80 ml) Massel Beef Style Liquid Stock

2 tsp Dijon mustard

0,048 gal (180 ml) pouring cream

21,2 oz (600 g) steamed cauliflower, coarsely chopped

5,3 oz (150 g) fresh green beans, steamed

Fresh continental parsley leaves, coarsely chopped, to serve

The preparation:

- Combine the beef, egg, shallot, parsley, garlic, allspice and nutmeg in a large bowl. Season well

- Roll tablespoonfuls of the mixture into balls

- Heat the oil in a large non-stick frying pan over medium-high heat. Cook the meatballs, turning often, for 6-8 minutes or until golden and just cooked through & transfer to a plate

- Add the stock, mustard and 0,033 gal (125 ml) cream to the pan and bring to the boil. Reduce heat and simmer for 5 minutes or until reduced by half

- Return the meatballs to the pan and simmer for 1-2 minutes or until heated through

- Place the cauliflower and remaining cream in a food processor and process until smooth

- Divide the cauliflower mash among serving plates. Top with the beans, meatballs and sauce. Serve scattered with parsley.

KETO CHICKEN PARMI BOWL

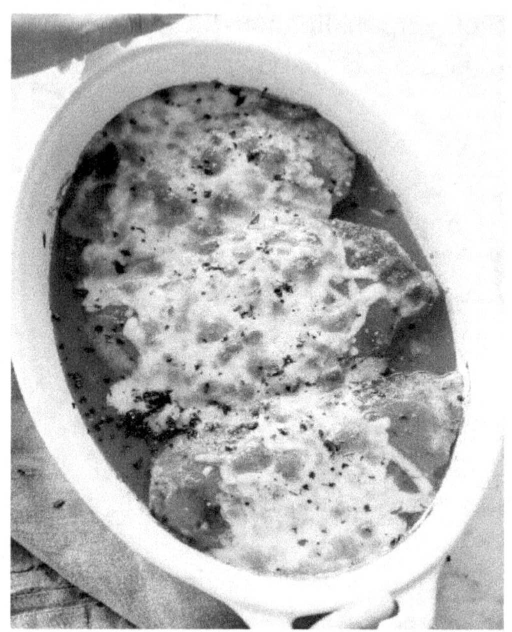

Ingredients:

1 egg

2,8 oz (80 g) almond meal

1,4 oz (40 g) finely grated parmesan

2 tsp finely chopped fresh continental parsley, plus extra to serve

4 x (about 4,4 oz (125 g) each) chicken breast schnitzels (uncrumbed)

Extra virgin olive oil, to shallow fry, plus extra to drizzle

0,021 gal (80 ml) tomato pasta sauce

4 slices smoked ham

1,8 oz (50 g) coarsely grated fresh mozzarella

2,2 lb (1 kg) - 1 head - cauliflower, trimmed, cut into florets

0,88 oz (25 g) butter

0,033 gal (125 ml) thickened cream

White pepper, to season

1 tsp chopped fresh chives, optional

The preparation:

- Lightly whisk the egg in a shallow bowl

- Combine the almond meal, parmesan and parsley on a plate.

- Dip 1 chicken piece in the egg, then into the almond meal mixture, pressing to coat. Transfer to a lined tray. Repeat with the remaining chicken, egg and almond meal mixture → Place in the fridge for 30 minutes to rest

- For the puree, place the cauliflower in a medium saucepan over high heat and cover with water. Cook for 15 – 20 minutes or until tender. Drain into a colander and set apart, reserving 1/3 cup of the cooking liquid

- Heat the butter in the saucepan over medium heat until foaming → add the cooked cauliflower, cream and reserved cooking liquid. Simmer for 3 minutes

-   Remove from the heat and use a stab blender to blend until smooth. Season with salt and white pepper. Stir through the chives, if using. Cover and set aside.

-   Heat 1cm of oil in a large, heavy based frypan over high heat. Cook the chicken in batches for 3 minutes on each side or until crisp and golden → transfer the chicken to the tray

-   Preheat the grill to high. Spoon a dollop of tomato pasta sauce over each chicken peace. Top with ham and sprinkle with cheese

-   Grill for 3-4 minutes or until the cheese is golden. Sprinkle with extra parsley if desired

-   Meanwhile, return the cauliflower puree to medium heat and cook, stirring for 2 minutes or until heated through. Serve the chicken with the puree.

KETO PANCAKES

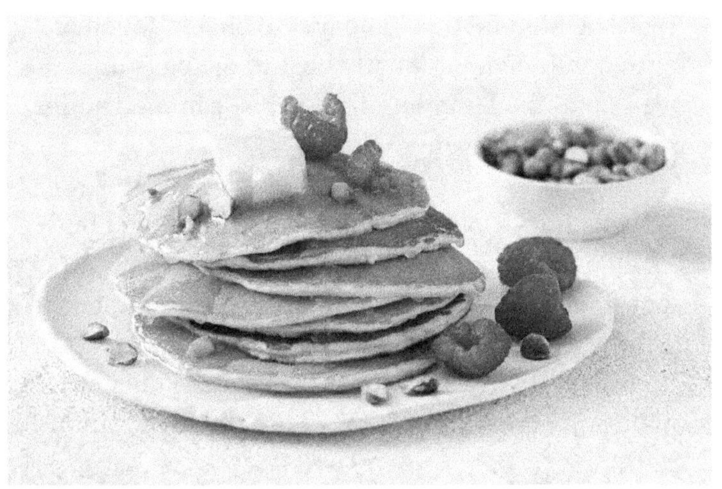

Ingredients:

2,8 oz (80 g) almond meal

4,4 oz (125 g) cream cheese, chopped, at room temperature

3 eggs

1 tsp vanilla extract

1/4 tsp baking powder

Melted butter, to cook

Butter, to serve

Chopped pistachios, to serve

Fresh raspberries, to serve (optional)

The preparation:

- Beat the almond meal and cream cheese together until combined. Gradually beat in the eggs until well combined and lump-free → stir in the vanilla and baking powder

- Brush a non-stick frying pan with the melted butter. Place over medium heat. Pour in about three 1/4 cup measures of the mixture and cook for 2 minutes or until golden. Carefully turn (the pancakes are a bit fragile) and cook for a further minute. Transfer to a plate and continue with the rest of the batter. Fun right?

Serve pancakes topped with butter, pistachios and raspberries, if using.

ONE-POT KETO ZUCCHINI ALFREDO

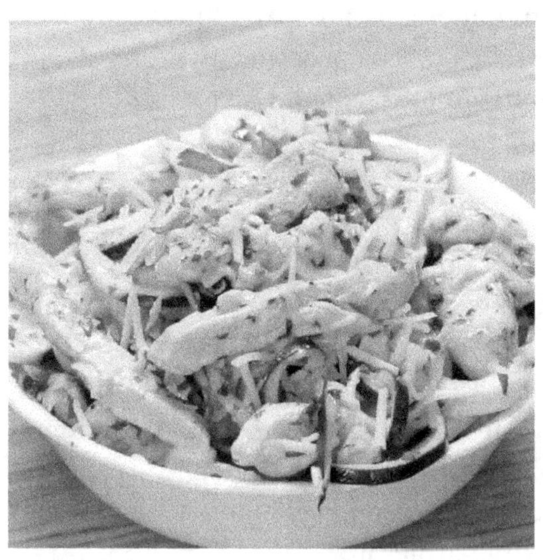

Ingredients:

1 tsp extra-virgin olive oil

0,53 oz (15 g) butter

2 x 8,8 oz (250 g) packets zucchini noodles

2 garlic cloves, finely chopped

3,5 oz (100 g) cream cheese, chopped

1 tsp thickened cream

0,7 oz (20 g) finely grated parmesan, (or vegetarian hard cheese) plus extra to serve

The preparation:

- Heat the oil and butter in a frying pan over medium-high heat until butter is foamy. Add the zucchini noodles. Use tongs to toss occasionally, for 1-2 minutes or until slightly wilted. Use tongs to transfer to a plate.

- Add the garlic to the pan. Cook, while stirring, for 1 minute or until aromatic. Add the cream cheese, cream and 0,016 gal (60 ml) water. Reduce heat to low

- Cook, stirring often, for 3 minutes or until mixture is smooth. Stir through the parmesan and season. Add the zucchini and use tongs to toss to combine. Serve with extra parmesan.

LOW-CARB KETO-FRIENDLY PIZZA

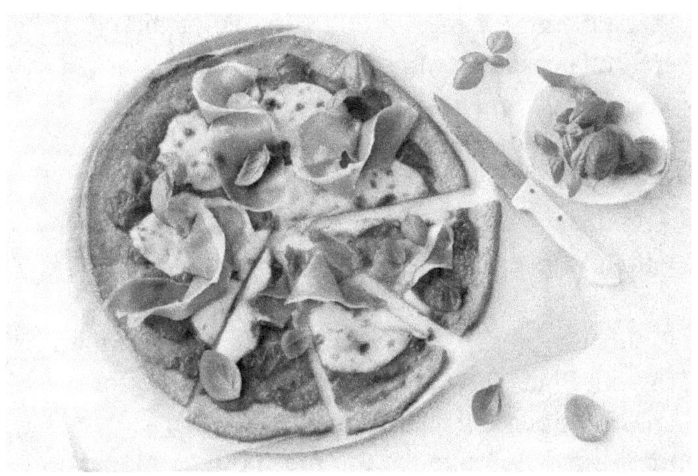

Ingredients:

4,9 oz (140 g) coarsely grated mozzarella

1,9 oz (55 g) almond meal

2 tsp cream cheese

1 egg

0,021 gal (80 ml) tomato pasta sauce

1,4 oz (40 g) sliced mozzarella

4 thin slices prosciutto

Fresh basil leaves, to serve

The preparation:

- Place the grated mozzarella, almond meal and cream cheese in a microwave-safe bowl. Microwave on HIGH (100%) for 1 minute, stirring halfway, or until melted and combined

- Add the egg and working quickly, beat vigorously with a wooden spoon until combined.

- Preheat oven to 392°F/356°F (200°C/180°C) fan forced. Place the 'dough' between 2 pieces of baking paper and roll to line a 12,6 inch (32 cm) pizza tray. Remove the top piece of baking paper and slide the dough with the bottom piece of baking paper onto the pizza tray → bake for 10 mins or until puffed and golden.

- Use the paper to slide the pizza from the tray. Flip back onto the tray to cook the other side. Cook for a further 5 minutes or until the top is golden

- Spread lightly with tomato pasta sauce and top with sliced mozzarella. Bake for 3-4 minutes or until the cheese has melted

- Drape with prosciutto and scatter with basil leaves.

KETO CLOUD BREAD

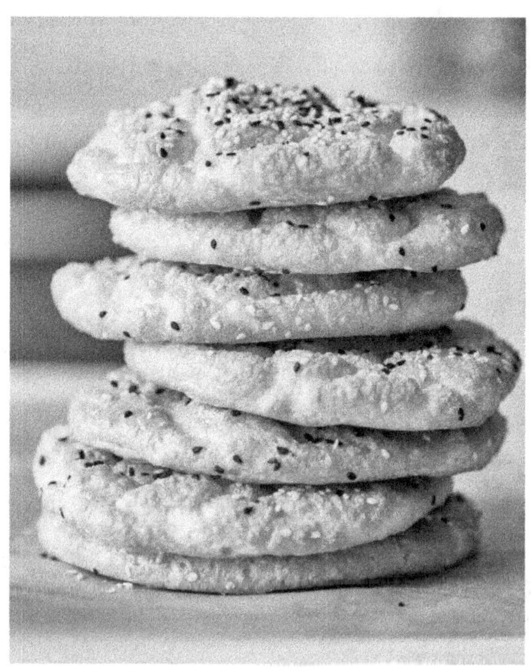

Ingredients:

3 eggs, separated

1/4 tsp cream of tartar

2,3 oz (65 g) crème fraiche

Pinch salt

1 tsp sesame seeds (optional)

The preparation:

- Preheat oven to 302°F/266°F (150°C/130°C) fan forced. Line two baking trays with baking paper

- Whisk the egg whites and cream of tartar in a bowl

- Meanwhile, whisk together the egg yolks, crème fraiche and salt in a small bowl until combined

- Add the egg yolk mixture into the egg white mixture and mix until combined

- Spoon two heaped dessert spoonful of the mixture onto the lined tray. Use the back of a spoon to spread slightly into an 3,15 inch (8 cm) disc. Repeat with the remaining mixture to create 8 discs. Sprinkle with sesame seeds, if using.

- Bake for 25-30 minutes or until golden. Now let them completely cool

KETO SNACK BARS

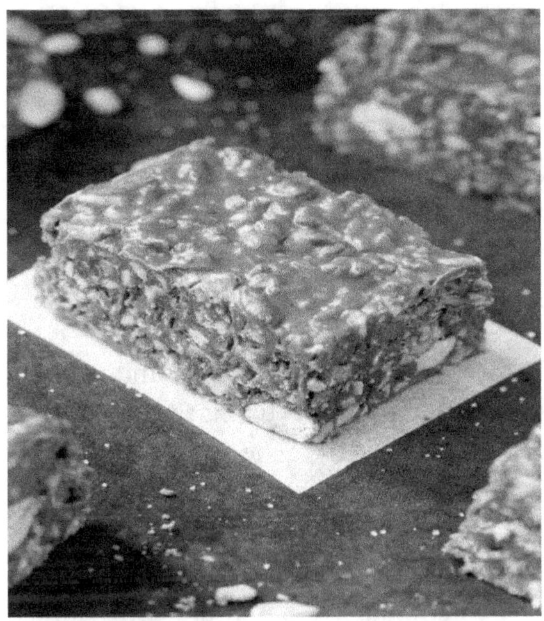

Ingredients:

3,0 oz (85 g) almonds

1,9 oz (55 g) walnut halves

2,8 oz (80 g) macadamia nuts

2,8 oz (80 g) pepitas

3,0 oz (85 g) desiccated coconut

1 tsp ground cinnamon

4,6 oz (130 g) peanut coconut spread

2,1 oz (60 g) solidified coconut oil

2 tsp vanilla bean paste

The preparation:

- Lightly grease and line a 6,3 x 10,24 inch (16 x 26 cm) (base measurement) lamington pan with baking paper

- Process the almonds, walnuts, macadamia nuts and pepitas in a food processor until coarsely chopped. Transfer to a large bowl → stir in the coconut and cinnamon

- Combine the peanut spread, coconut oil and vanilla in a small saucepan and cook, stirring, over low heat for 3-5 minutes or until melted and well combined

- Add the peanut mixture to the dry ingredients and mix until well combined. Press mixture firmly into prepared pan, smoothing surface with the back of a spoon

- Cover and place in the fridge for 2-3 hours or until firm. Cut into 16 bars

KETO CHICKEN COCONUT CURRY WITH BROCCOLI RICE

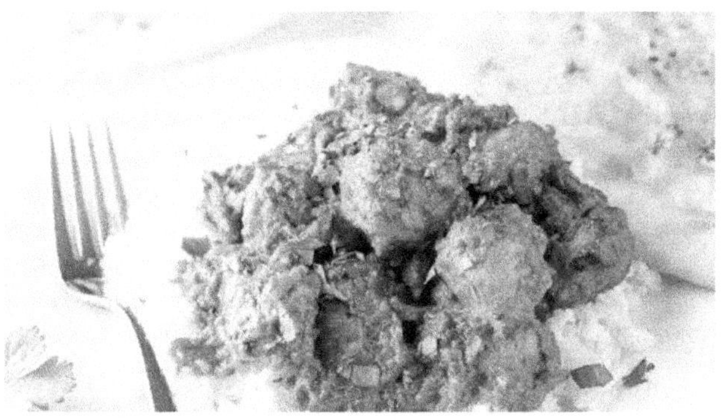

Ingredients:

2 tsp macadamia oil

21,2 oz (600 g) chicken thigh fillets, cut into 3cm pieces

1 brown onion, sliced

2 garlic cloves, crushed

2 tsp finely grated fresh ginger

2 long red chilies, finely chopped, plus extra sliced to serve

1/2 tsp turmeric

2 tsp brown mustard seeds

2 tsp ground cumin

1 tsp ground coriander

0,106 gal (400 ml) coconut cream

17,6 gal (500 g) broccoli, chopped

Lime juice, to taste

Fish sauce, to taste

3,5 oz (100 g) baby spinach leaves

The preparation:

- Heat half the oil in a large saucepan or wok over high heat. Add half the chicken and cook, stirring occasionally, for 2-3 minutes or until browned. Transfer to a plate & repeat with the remaining chicken and set the chicken apart

- Add the remaining oil and the onion to the pan. Cook stirring, for 3-4 minutes or until softened → add the garlic, ginger, chili, turmeric, mustard seeds, cumin and coriander & cook, stirring, for 2 minutes or until aromatic

- Add the coconut cream and the chicken. Bring to the boil. Partially cover and reduce heat to low. Simmer for 20 minutes or until the chicken is tender

- Meanwhile, process the broccoli in a food processor until finely chopped (like rice). Transfer the broccoli to a large microwave-safe bowl. Cover and microwave on HIGH for 2-3 minutes or until just tender

- Remove curry from heat and season with lime juice and fish sauce, to taste. Sprinkle with the spinach and extra chili and serve with the broccoli

KETO FISH AND CHIPS

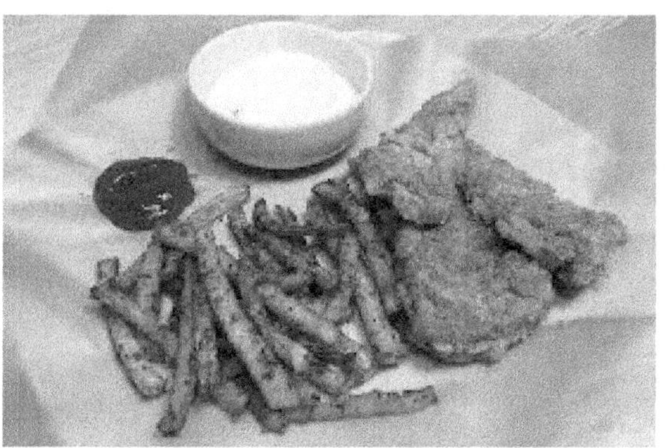

Ingredients:

2 eggs

1 tsp pouring cream

5,5 oz (155 g) almond meal

1,4 oz (40 g) finely grated parmesan cheese

1 large lemon, rind finely grated

1/3 cup chopped fresh continental parsley

1 tsp dried chili flakes (optional)

2 avocados

2 large zucchinis, cut into long wedges

4 x 4,4 oz (125 g) skinless firm white fish fillets

0,021 gal (80 ml) rice bran oil

Mixed salad leaves, to serve

Lemon wedges, to serve

The preparation:

- Preheat oven to 428°F/392°F (220°C/200°C) fan forced. Line a large baking tray with baking paper

- Whisk the eggs, cream and 1 tbs water together in a large shallow bowl

- Combine the almond meal, cheese, rind, parsley and chili flakes (if using) in a shallow bowl

- Halve each avocado, remove stone, peel away skin and cut each into 6-8 wedges.

- Working with 1 piece at a time, coat a piece of avocado in the egg mixture, allowing excess to drip off, then coat in the almond meal mixture. Repeat with the zucchini and fish

- Crumb the avocado and zucchini and spread evenly over the prepared tray

- Place the fish on a plate, cover and place in the fridge for 10 minutes to rest

- Spray the crumbed avocado and zucchini generously with oil. Bake for a couple of minutes

- Heat the oil in a large non-stick frying pan over medium-high heat. Cook the fish for 2-3 minutes each side or until golden and crisp. Serve fish and chips with salad leaves and lemon wedges

KETO STRAWBERRY, ALMOND AND CHOCOLATE MUFFINS

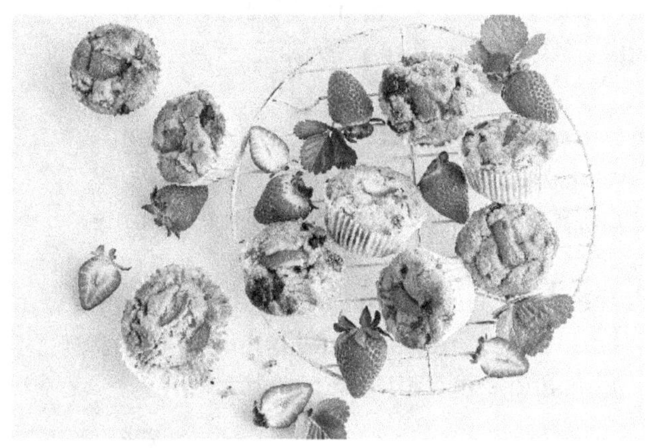

Ingredients:

0,88 oz (25 g) coconut flour

3 tsp baking powder

7,1 oz (200 g) almond meal

1,8 oz (50 g) powdered stevia sweetener

8,8 oz (250 g) strawberries, hulled, chopped

2,6 oz (75 g) dark chocolate (85% cocoa), chopped

3 eggs, lightly whisked

2 tsp vanilla extract

0,016 gal (60 ml) almond milk

4,4 oz (125 g) unsalted butter, melted

The preparation:

- Preheat oven to 338°F/302°F (170°C/150°C) fan forced. Line 12 holes of an 0,021 gal (80 ml) capacity muffin pan with paper cases

- Sift the coconut flour and baking powder into a large bowl. Add the almond meal, stevia, strawberries and chocolate and stir to combine

- Whisk the eggs, vanilla and almond milk together in a jug. Add the egg mixture and butter to the dry ingredients and stir until just combined.

- Divide the mixture among the prepared muffin holes. Bake for 20-25 minutes or until golden and a skewer inserted into the centre comes out clean. Set aside for 5 minutes, to cool, before transferring to a wire rack to cool completely

AVOCADO AND CUCUMBER SALAD

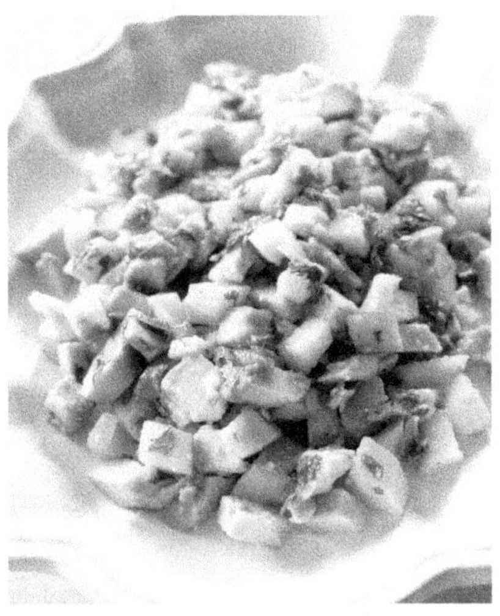

Ingredients:

6,2 oz (175 g) baby salad leaves

2 medium avocados, chopped

4 green onions, thinly sliced

2 Lebanese cucumbers, halved, thinly sliced

1/4 cup lemon juice

1/4 cup olive oil

The preparation:

- Prepare the ingredients like mentioned in the recipes list.

-   Combine the salad leaves, avocado, onion and
    cucumber in a bowl

-   Mix the lemon juice and oil with the salad and
    season with salt

AVOCADO, SPINACH AND WALNUT SALAD

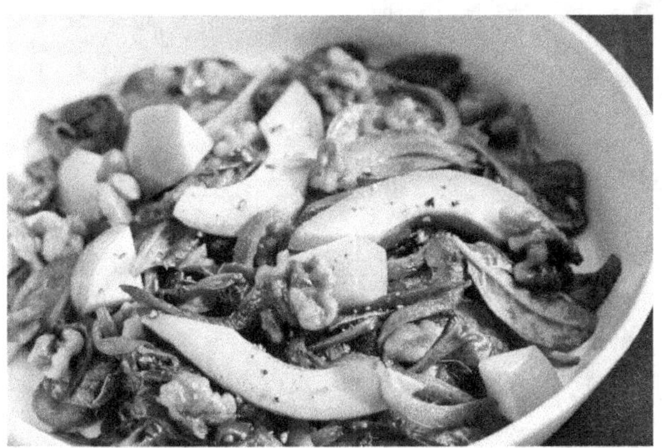

Ingredients:

1 1/2 tbs roughly choppcd walnuts

7,1 oz (200 g) baby spinach leaves

1 ripe avocado, peeled, stone removed, sliced

Juice of 1 lemon

The preparation:

- Place walnuts into a small frying pan. Cook over medium heat, shaking frying pan often, for 3 to 4 minutes or until walnuts are golden and roasted. Remove from heat

- Arrange spinach and avocado on serving plates. Sprinkle over walnuts. Drizzle with lemon juice. Season with salt and pepper & serve

EASY KETO CHICKEN CHOW MIEN

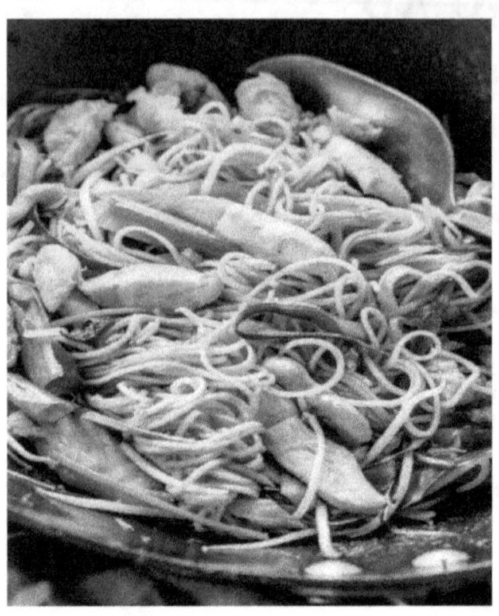

Ingredients:

2 tbs peanut oil

17,6 oz (500 g) chicken thigh fillets, thinly sliced

8,8 oz (250 g) broccoli, cut into florets

4 garlic cloves, thinly sliced

1 long fresh red chili, deseeded, finely chopped

extra fresh chili, finely chopped, to serve

1/4 small red cabbage, sliced

8,8 oz (250 g) zucchini noodles

3,9 oz (110 g) trimmed bean sprouts

2,5 oz (75 g) roasted unsalted cashew nuts

2 tbs gluten-free soy sauce

2 tsp sesame oil

Fresh coriander sprigs, to serve

The preparation:

- Heat half the peanut oil in a large wok over high heat. Stir-fry half the chicken for 2-3 minutes or until golden & transfer to a plate. Repeat with remaining chicken

- Heat the remaining peanut oil in the wok when finished with the chicken. Stir-fry the broccoli, garlic and chili for 2 minutes or until tender crisp. Add the cabbage and zucchini noodles. Stir-fry for 1 minute or until just tender

- Return the chicken to the wok along with the bean sprouts, cashews, soy sauce and sesame oil. Stir-fry for 1 minute and mix everything

- Serve sprinkled with coriander and extra chili

SEA BREAM CEVICHE WITH CITRUS OIL

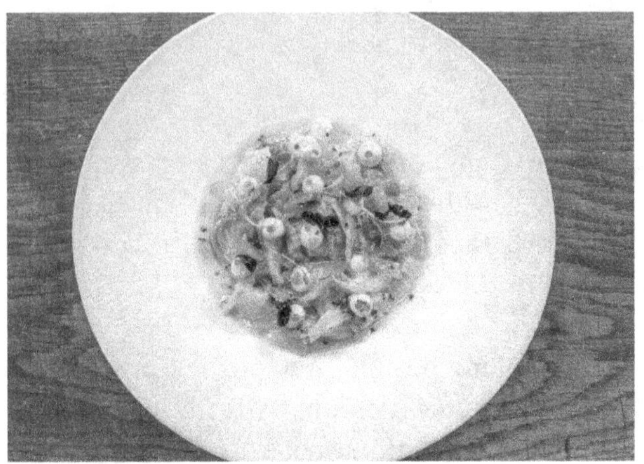

Ingredients:

5,3 oz (150 g) sea bream

2 tsp olive oil

1/2 shallot

15 coriander leaves

The juice of half an untreated lemon + zest

Untreated of half an orange juice + zest

Salt & pepper

The preparation:

- To make this ceviche recipe, start by finely chopping the half shallot and then chop the coriander

- Wash and squeeze half the lemon and half the orange & take the citrus zest

- Then cut the sea bream into 1cm cubes. Place in a bowl and cover it with the citrus juice and the shallot, coriander and olive oil as well as the zest. Salt and pepper to your liking
    - Be careful to dose the zest according to your tastes to prevent the dish from being too strong

- Cover and leave to stand in the refrigerator for 1 to 2 hours so the citrus juice penetrates the fish

- Finally, coarsely drain the fish to get rid of a little excess citrus juice and now you have a very fresh ceviche

AVOCADO AND PEPPER OMELET

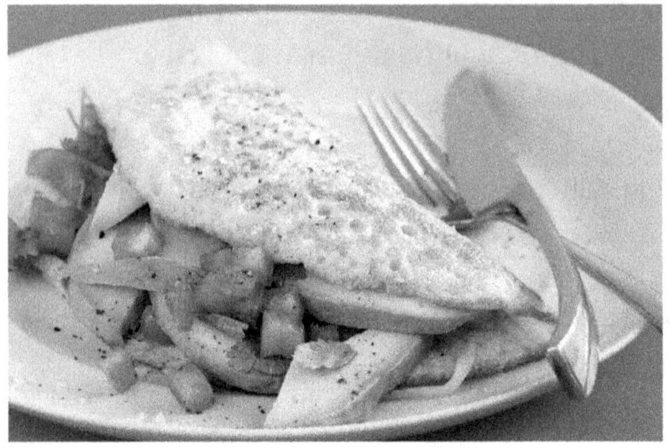

Ingredients:

2 organic eggs

1 avocado

1 tomato

½ minced onion

1 chopped bell pepper

Salt and pepper

2 tsp of coconut oil

The preparation:

- Heat 2 teaspoons of coconut oil and add the eggs → add the onions and chopped peppers

- Garnish your omelet with the avocado and the tomato (which are both cut in small squares)

PEANUT BUTTER YOGURT AND COCOA

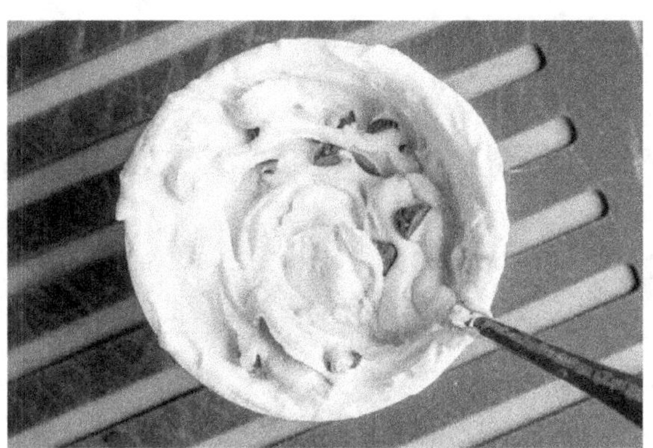

Ingredients:

8,8 oz (250 g) sugar-free yogurt

½ tbs peanut butter

1 tsp cocoa powder

½ tsp stevia

The preparation:

- Mix the yogurt with the peanut butter, cocoa powder and stevia. Simple and enjoyable

EGGS WITH CHEESE, SALAMI AND SPINACH

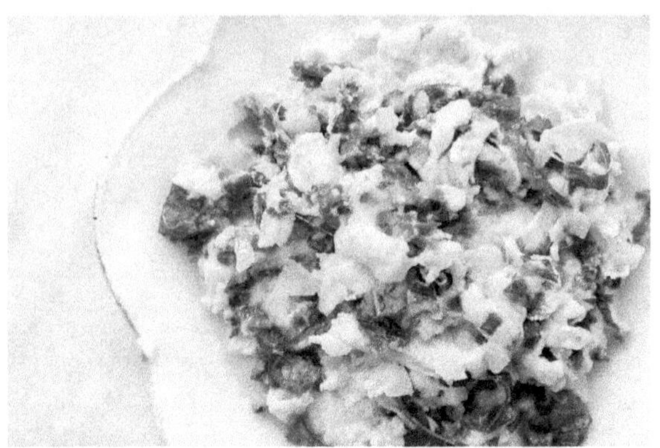

Ingredients:

2 eggs

Salt and pepper

Grated cheese

3 slices of salami

5,3 oz (150 g) fresh spinach

The preparation:

- Heat 2 teaspoons of coconut oil and add the eggs →
  add pepper and salt to taste

- Cut the salami into small pieces and add the salami
  and grated cheese to the eggs

- Garnish with 5,3 oz (150 g) of fresh spinach

HAZELNUTS, CELERY STICKS AND CREAM CHEESE

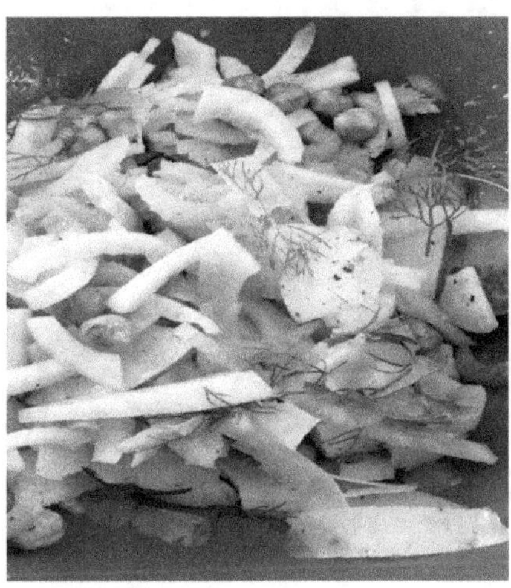

Ingredients:

A handful of hazelnuts

6 celery sticks

3 tbs cream cheese

The preparation:

- Cut the celery sticks into very small pieces and to the same with the hazelnuts and the cream cheese

- Mix everything and enjoy!

BEEF WITH VEGETABLES

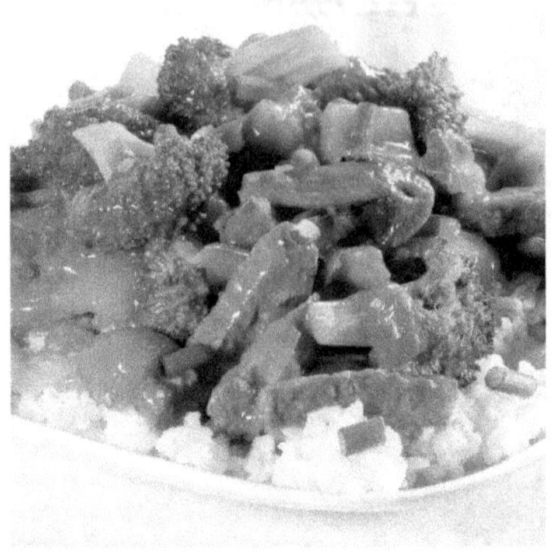

Ingredients:

7,1 oz (200 g) beef cutlet

8,8 oz (250 g) frozen vegetables

2 tsp of coconut oil

The preparation:

- Thaw the vegetables

- Heat 2 teaspoons of coconut oil and brown the beef cutlet in a pan

- Cook the vegetables according to your taste.

TUNA WITH VEGETABLES

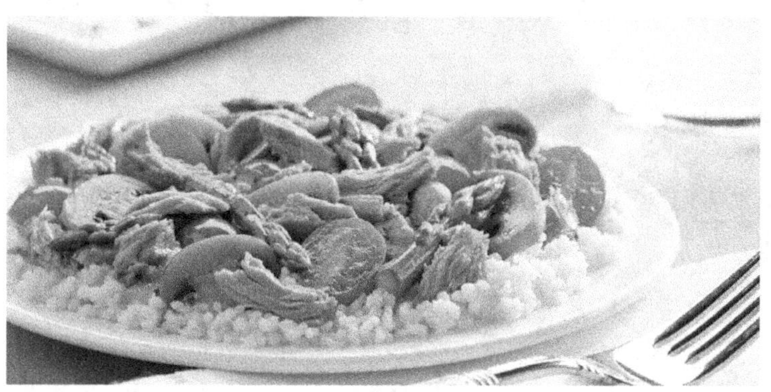

Ingredients:

4,4 oz (125 g) canned tuna in oil

7,1 oz (200 g) frozen vegetables

1 tbs mayonnaise

The preparation:

- Thaw the vegetables

- Cook the vegetables according to your taste

- Remove the tuna from the box and place it on a plate

- Add 1 tablespoons mayonnaise to the tuna

- Add the vegetables and mix well

CHICKEN WITH PESTO, VEGETABLES AND FRESH CHEESE

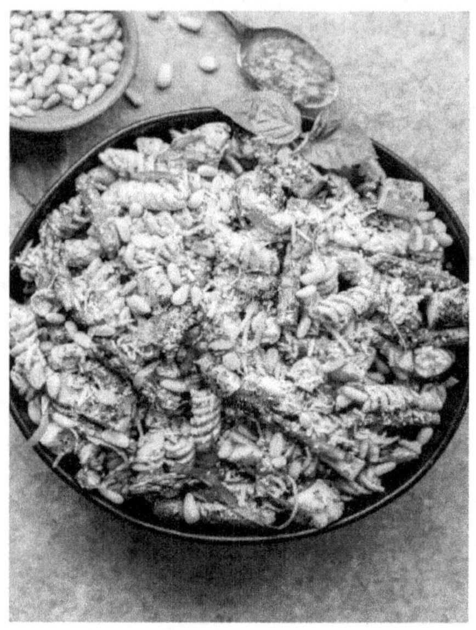

Ingredients:

10,6 oz (300 g) chicken

1 tbs pesto

1 tomato

A sachet of sautéed vegetable

A bowl of cream cheese to your liking

The preparation:

- Cook the chicken and cover with pesto on both sides

- Cook the vegetables to your liking

- Cut the chicken into pieces, add the vegetables and tomato & mix

- Add fresh cheese to your liking

MAYONNAISE MINCED STEAKS

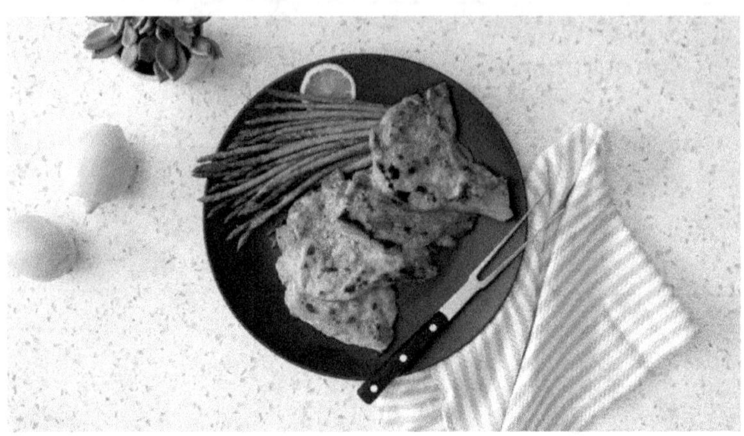

Ingredients:

2 ground beef steak

0,011 gal (40 ml) mayonnaise (optional)

1 tbs olive oil

The preparation:

- Heat 1 tablespoon olive oil and cook the minced steaks

- Serve with mayonnaise (optional)

EGGS WITH SALMON AND SPINACH

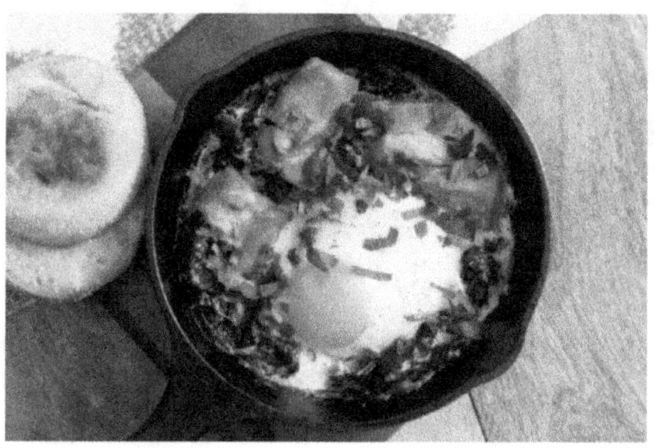

Ingredients:

15,9 oz (450 g) frozen leeks with cream

14,1 oz (400 g) pink salmon

4 eggs

1 tsp of herbs of your choice

½ red pepper

The preparation:

- Preheat the oven to 347°F (175 ° C)

- Cut all the ingredients to small pieces

- Mix all the ingredients

- Pour into muffin tins, almost to the edge

- Bake for about 15 minutes

RASPBERRY CHIA SEED PUDDING

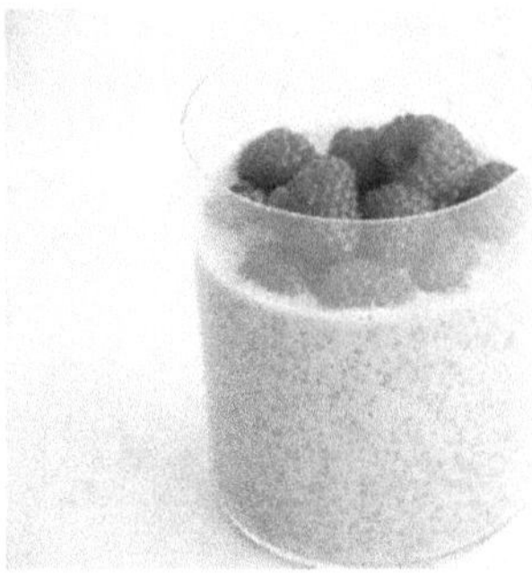

Ingredients:

Unsweetened coconut milk – 4,2 oz (120 g)

Chia seeds – 1,4 oz (40 g)

Frozen raspberries – 2,1 oz (60 g)

Erythritol / Stevia – 0,35 oz (10 g)

Few drops of cinnamon/vanilla extract/orange blossom

The preparation:

- Mix the coconut milk and the chia seeds. Flavor with cinnamon, a few drops of vanilla extract or orange blossom

- Reserve in the fridge for 2 hours

- Meanwhile thaw the raspberries

- Add the raspberries over the pudding, sprinkle with stevia / erythritol sweetener. if necessary and enjoy

BULLET PROOF COFFEE

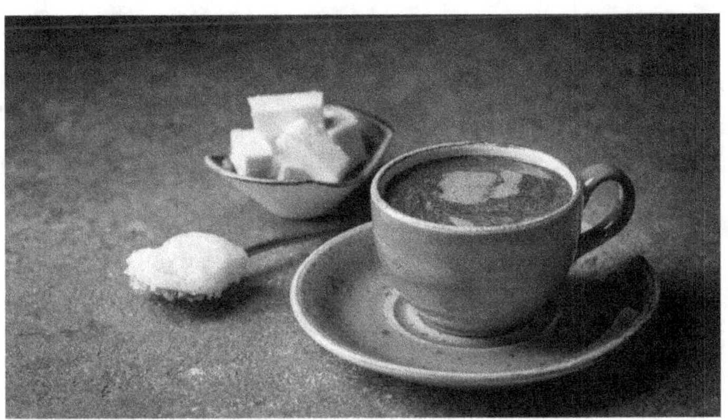

Ingredients:

Black coffee – 7,1 oz (200 g)

Coconut oil – 0,35 oz (10 g)

Sweet butter – 0,7 oz (20 g)

The preparation:

- Run a large black coffee

- In a shaker, mix the coffee with the butter and the coconut oil

- Sweeten if necessary, with a sweetener like Stevia

MIXED KETO SALAD

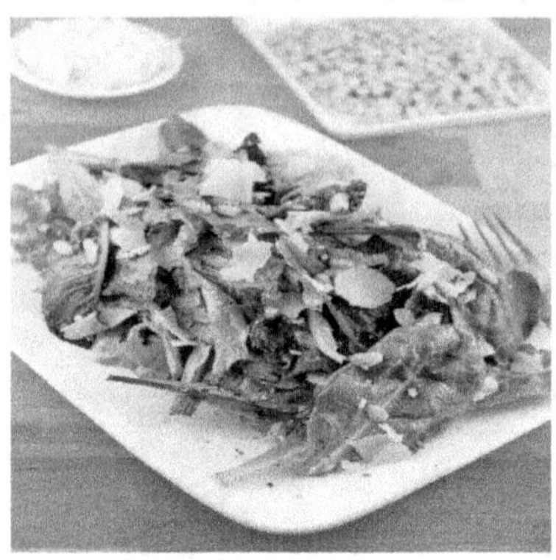

Ingredients:

Young shoot salad – 3,5 oz (100 g)

Roast chicken, cooked – 1,8 oz (50 g)

Cucumber – 3,5 oz (100 g) (1/2 cucumber)

Tomatoes – 1,8 oz (50 g) (2 small tomatoes)

Hard-boiled egg – 3,5 oz (100 g) (3 eggs)

Avocado - 3,5 oz (100 g) (1/2 avocado)

Crespo black olives – 1,8 oz (50 g)

Olive oil – 1,8 oz (50 g)

The preparation:

- Cut out the ingredients & mix with olive oil and season to taste

- You can vary the ingredients

KETOGENIC ZUCCHINI SOUP

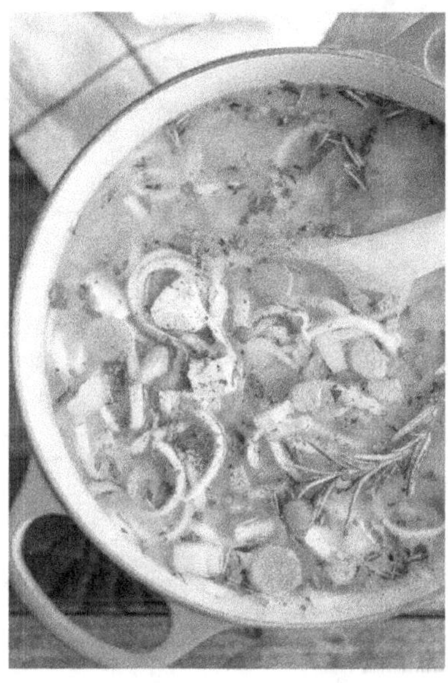

Ingredients:

Courgette – 3,5 oz (100 g) (1/2 courgette)

Thick fresh cream 30% - 2,1 oz (60 g)

Dijon mustard – 0,35 oz (10 g)

The preparation:

- Blanch the sliced zucchini in boiling water for 10 minutes

- Mix with the crème fraiche and mustard

- Season and serve

SAVORY MUFFINS AND SWEET MUFFINS

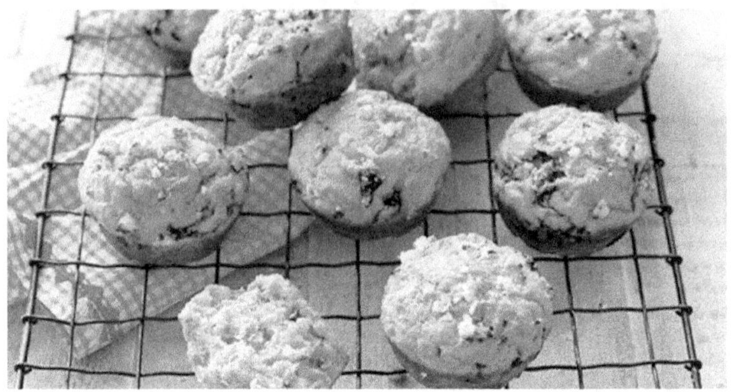

Ingredients:

4,4 oz (125 g) mascarpone

4 eggs

1 tsp coffee xanthan gum

2 tbs flour coconut

2 tbs almond flour

2 tbs cocoa powder (unsweetened!)

1 tsp coffee baking powder

1/2 tsp coffee baking soda

2 tbs coconut oil

2 tbs butter

sweetener to taste

The preparation:

- Mix all the dry ingredients: xanthan gum, coconut and almond flour, yeast, cocoa, yeast, bicarbonate

- Add the 4 eggs one by one, and beat for 1 to 2 minutes with an electric whisk (this is important because the xanthan gum, emulsified, will make your dough elastic and therefore allow you to obtain super soft muffins)

- Add the mascarpone, the melted butter, the coconut oil and the sweetener and beat again until a homogeneous paste is obtained

- Divide among muffin tins and put in the oven for 35 to 45 minutes in a medium oven (356 ° F/180 ° C), monitoring the cooking

OLIVE CAKE

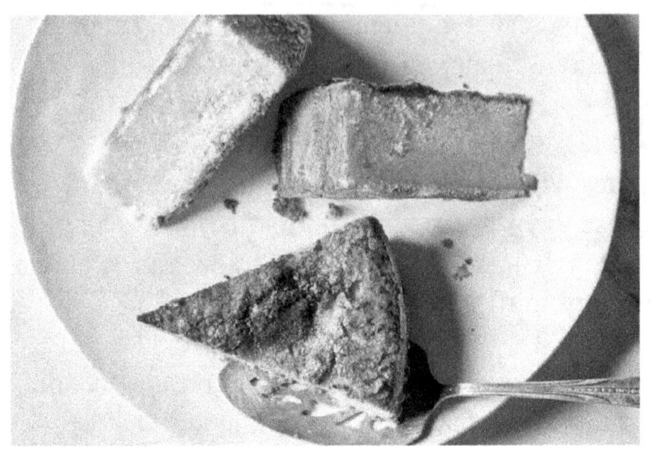

Ingredients:

4,4 oz (125 g) mascarpone

4 eggs

3 tbs soup powder almond

1 tbs flour coconut

1 tsp coffee baking powder

7,1 oz (200 g) grated cheese

7,1 oz (200 g) pitted green olives

7,1 oz (200 g) garlic sausage

salt and pepper

The preparation:

- Strongly mix the eggs and the mascarpone with a whisk

- Add the almond, coconut flours, the yeast, salt and pepper & beat again to obtain a homogeneous dough

- Cut the sausage into cubes and add it to the preparation with the grated cheese and the pitted green olives

- Mix with a spatula to integrate the ingredients well and pour into a mold (if you use the Omnia oven, the silicone mold is ideal!).

- Bake over medium heat (356 ° F/180 ° C) for 45 to 50 minutes (watch for baking, the cake should be nicely browned on top)

EGGPLANT CAVIAR

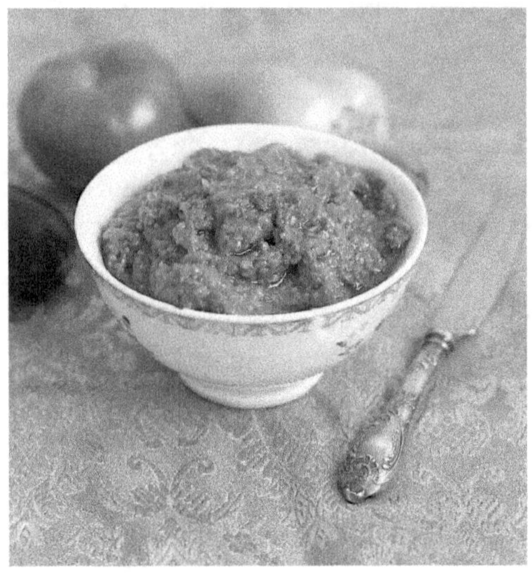

Ingredients:

2 eggplants

2 garlic cloves

1/2 lemon

2 tbs olive oil

Salt and pepper

The preparation:

- Wash the eggplants, cut the peduncle and prick them with a fork.

- Arrange in a suitable dish and cook for 8-10 minutes in the microwave, maximum power

-   Open the cooked eggplants and collect the flesh
    with a spoon

-   Put the flesh, the peeled garlic cloves, the oil, the
    salt, the pepper and the juice of half a lemon in the
    blender (I use a hand blender, but a blender does the
    job just as well)

-   Blend until a creamy texture is obtained. And now,
    it only remains to put it in the fridge

HOMEMADE CREAM CHEESE COTTAGE

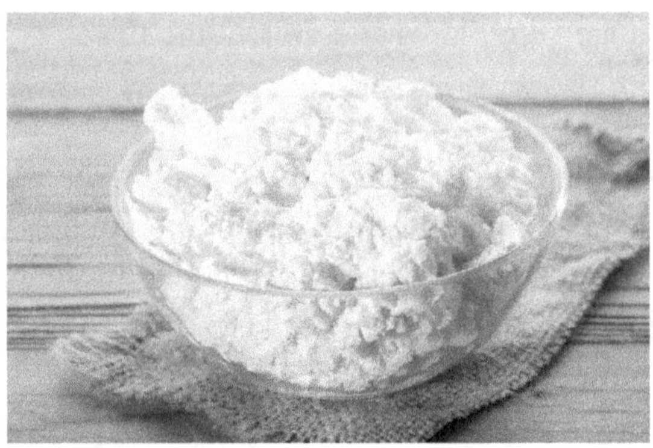

Ingredients:

0,26 gal (1 liter) Whole milk (preferably fresh)

0,005 gal (2 cl) Vinegar (preferably white, but works with classic wine vinegar)

0,005 gal (2 cl) water

1 tsp salt

2 tbs heavy cream

Ingredients to your liking for taste: chocolate/cheese/vanilla

The preparation:

-    Bring the milk to a boil in a heavy-bottomed saucepan

-    Combine water, vinegar and salt in a small container (+ your own addition)
-    Once the milk is simmering, and leaving the pan on the heat, over medium heat, mix gently with a large spoon, dripping the vinegar water

- Add the thick cream and mix gently

- Transfer to an airtight container and cool quickly. It
  will stay their 4-5 days without problem

ZUCCHINI CROQUETTES

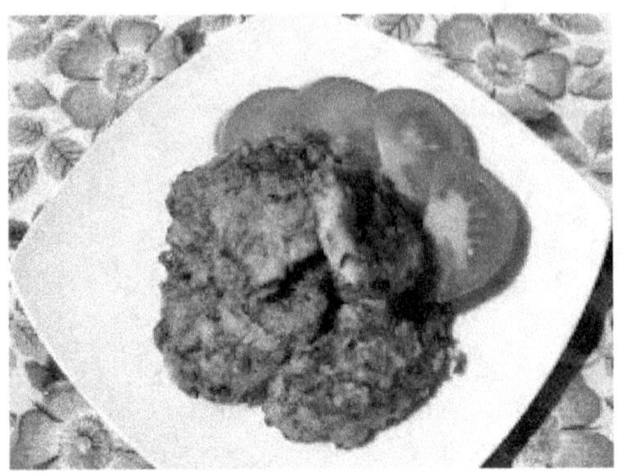

Ingredients:

3,5 oz (100 g) grated zucchini

2 eggs

1,2 oz (35 g) grated parmesan

0,7 oz (20 g) almond powder

0,35 oz (10 g) coconut flour

olive oil

The preparation:

- Mix the eggs with the almond powder, parmesan and coconut flour

- Add the zucchini, previously grated and carefully wrung out

- Cook in a small pile in an oiled pan previously heated over medium heat, 4-5 minutes per side

CHEESE-HERRING SALAD

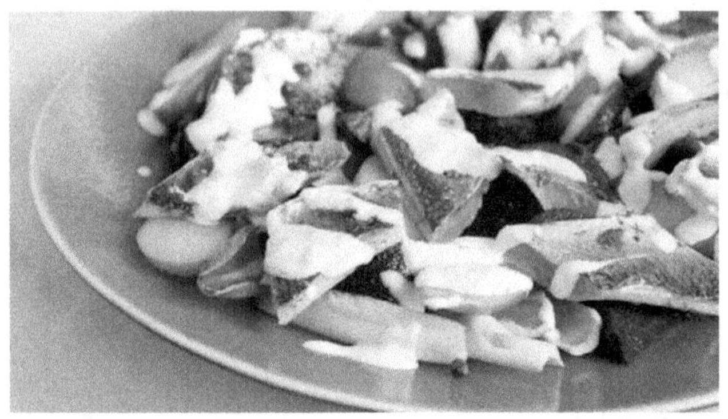

Ingredients:

1 lettuce salad bag

1 packet smoked herring (preferably sweet)

2 tbs olive oil

1/2 red onion

The preparation:

- Mince the onion and cut the herring into thin strips

- Mix all the ingredients & lightly peppering

FISH BREAD

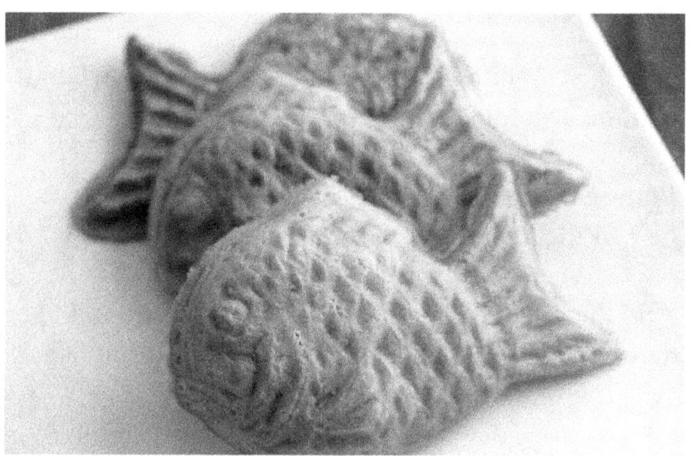

Ingredients:

2,2 lb (1 kg) white hake and cod fish (frozen or fresh)

0,053 gal (20 cl) liquid cream

court bouillon

1 cooked leek

2 eggs

1 tbs chopped parsley

salt and pepper

The preparation:

- Put the fish in a pot filled with cold salted water with the court bouillon

- As soon as the water boils, cook for barely 5 minutes, drain thoroughly and mash with a fork

-   Mix the cream, eggs, salt and pepper in a bowl and
    add the crumbled fish

-   Pour half of the dough into a cake mold and place
    half of the leek over the entire length

-   Add the chopped parsley to the rest of the dough
    and now fill the mold with the remaining dough and
    cover with the rest of the leek

-   Cover with buttered aluminum foil and bake in a
    bain-marie for about 1 hour at 356 ° F (180 ° C)

-   Unmold out of the oven and keep cool. Decorate
    just before serving if you want

CHARD OMELETT

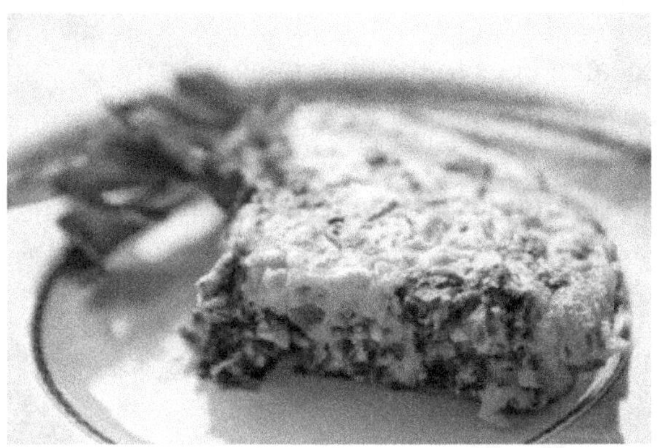

Ingredients:

1 bouquet of young chard

1 garlic clove

4 eggs

3 tbs olive oil

Salt and pepper

The preparation:

-   Remove the ribs and wash the chard with plenty of
    water. Wring them out and coarsely chop them with
    a knife

-   Heat the olive oil over medium heat in a pan

-   Put the chard in the pan and cover. Cook for 10-12
    minutes over medium heat, stirring occasionally

- Beat 4 eggs, a clove of chopped garlic, salt and pepper

- Add the beaten eggs to the chard, taking care to empty the pan of water returned by the chard

- Cook for 5-6 minutes. I usually fold mine like a pancake to form a thick rectangle, easier to cut into cubes

COCONUT KETO CURRY SHRIMP

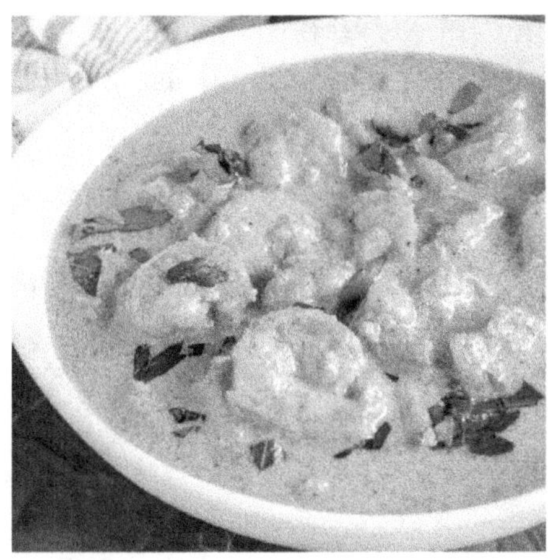

Ingredients:

21,2 oz (600 g) Raw shrimps

4 tbs coconut oil

1 clove garlic, minced

2 tbs chopped onion

1 tbs chopped fresh ginger

1 tbs red curry paste (radius world cuisine)

0,066 gal (25 cl) of coconut milk

Salt & pepper

2 small zucchinis

The preparation:

- Heat the coconut oil in a heavy-bottomed pan, and add the chopped garlic, onion and ginger. Heat over high heat, mixing for a few minutes.

- Add the peeled shrimp and the red curry paste, and sear over high heat 2-3 minutes, sautéing the shrimp regularly so that they soak up the sauce

- Add the coconut milk, salt and pepper. Reduce heat and cover to simmer

- Cut the zucchini into thin strips with a peeler or a spiralizer and add them to the shrimp. Raise the heat, mix again

- Simmer for a few minutes over low heat and serve.
    - You could serve it with konjac rice and fresh chopped cilantro

EGG KEFTA

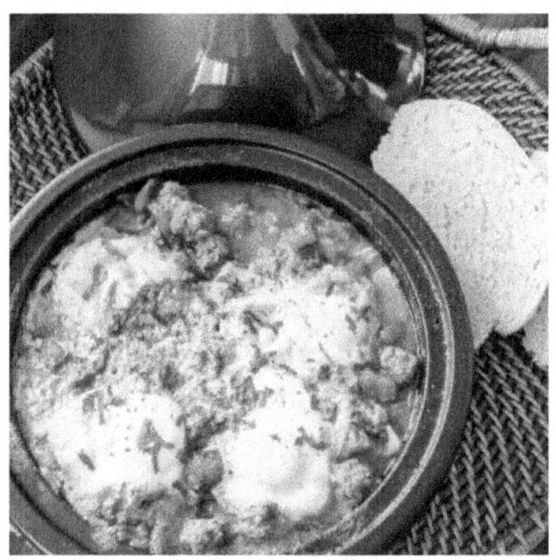

Ingredients:

14,1 oz (400 g) Ground beef

1/2 white onion, thinly sliced

1/2 tsp coffee Garlic powder

2 tbs soup Mix spice kofta (coriander, cumin, paprika essentially)

7,1 oz (200 g) Crushed tomatoes

4 eggs

4 tsp olive oil

Salt, pepper and fresh coriander

The preparation:

- In a bowl, mix the ground meat, garlic powder, kofta spices, minced onion, salt, pepper and 1 tsp olive oil

- Form 8 meatballs and brown over high heat in a heavy skillet

- When the meatballs are golden on all sides, pour the crushed tomatoes, bring to the boil and then reduce for 10 to 15 minutes over medium heat

- Turn the meatballs so that they are well soaked in the sauce and break the eggs in the sauce between the meatballs

- Cover and simmer over low heat for about ten minutes

- Serve with coarsely chopped fresh cilantro

MEATLOAF

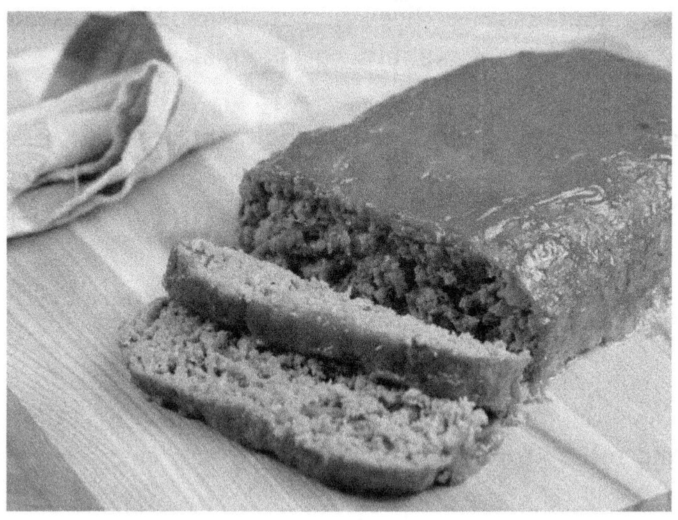

Ingredients:

17,6 oz (500 g) minced meat

1 yellow onion

1 garlic clove

1 egg

1,1 oz (30 g) melted butter

1,1 oz (30 g) fresh cheese (Philadelphia type)

5,3 oz (150 g) grated cheese (I used cheddar for this first try)

12 smoked breast slices

Oregano, salt and pepper

The preparation:

- Arrange the breast slices on a cellophane sheet, overlapping them slightly so as to make a plate

- Finely chop the onion and garlic with a knife

- Mix all the ingredients with a spoon
    - o avoid mixing in a food processor or kneading for too long, the result would be too dense

- Place the meat mixture on the smoked breast 'carpet' and roll up to form a loaf

- Bake in a suitable dish for 45 minutes at 392 ° F (200 ° C)

CURRY COCONUT SQUASH SOUP

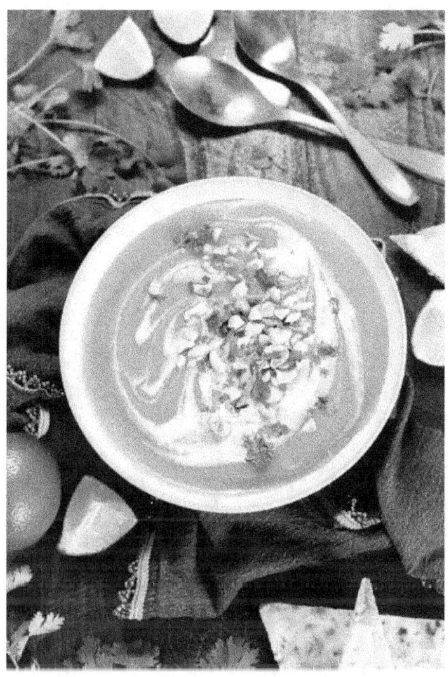

Ingredients:

4,4 lb (2 kg) squash (it is possible to use different squashes, pumpkin, butternut, pumpkin, etc.)

2 cans of coconut milk (about 28,2 oz/800g)

1 tbs curry powder

salt and pepper

olive oil

The preparation:

- Cut the squash in half and remove the seeds with a spoon

- Brush with a little olive oil and bake in the oven 90 minutes at 356 ° F (180 ° C)

- Let the squash cool before spooning the flesh

- Place the flesh of the squash in a pan with the coconut milk and the curry. Salt, pepper and mix

- Reheat on low heat and enjoy!

COCONUT CHICKEN SOUP

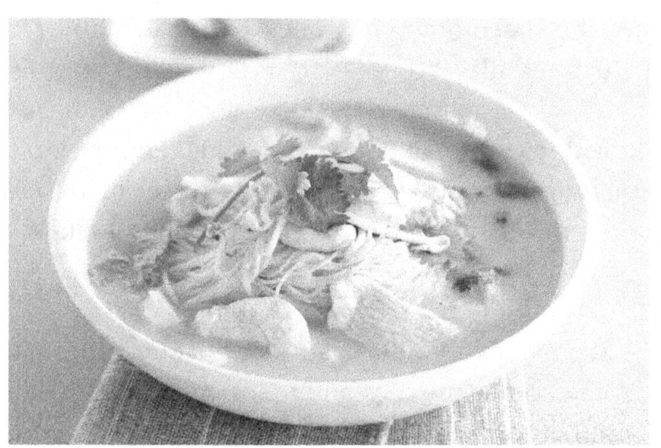

Ingredients:

2 chicken breasts

1 small zucchini

1/2 onion

1 packet konjac noodles

4 tbs coconut oil

1 tsp coffee red curry paste (the radius cuisines)

1 coconut cream briquette

chopped fresh cilantro

1 glass of broth (or water with a cube broth added)

Salt & pepper

The preparation:

- Brown the sliced onion in a thick-bottomed pan with coconut oil

- Add the curry paste and the whole chicken breasts, season with salt and pepper, pour in the broth and simmer until the meat can fray with a fork (it takes a good hour)

- Shred the meat with a fork, add the zucchini cut into strips, the konjac noodles and the coconut cream, and simmer again for 30 minutes

- Serve with a little chopped fresh cilantro

GINGERBREAD ROLLS

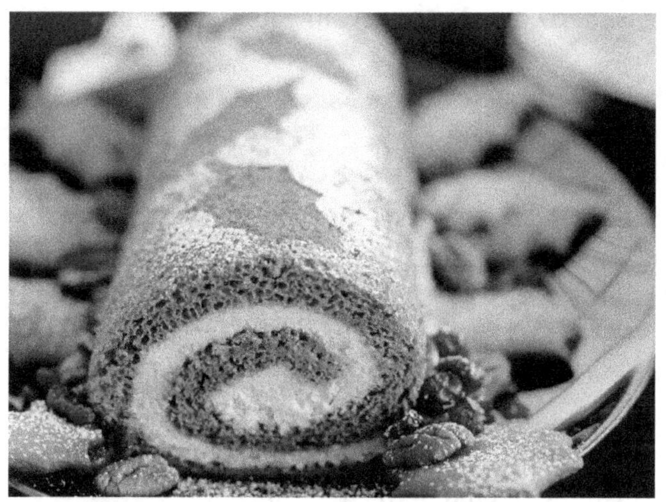

Ingredients:

2 eggs

4,2 oz (120 g) almond powder

2,8 oz (80 g) heavy cream

2,1 oz (60 g) erythritol powder

1,8 oz (50 g) melted butter

1,4 oz (40 g) of flax flour

3 tbs spice mixture in gingerbread

2 tbs psyllium

1 tsp coffee baking powder

The preparation:

- Whisk the eggs, heavy cream and melted butter

- Then add the sweetener, spices and baking powder and mix thoroughly

- Then gradually add the almond powder, flax flour and psyllium, taking care to have a homogeneous mixture

- Reserve 15 minutes in the fridge before making small walnut-sized balls

- Preheat the oven to 356 ° F (180 ° C)

- Place the balls on a baking sheet covered with parchment paper, flattening them slightly

- Bake 15 to 18 minutes (a toothpick planted in a cookie should come out dry)

- Let cool before decorating with 85% melted chocolate and / or hazelnuts (optional)

KETO CHOCOLATE & PEANUT CAKE

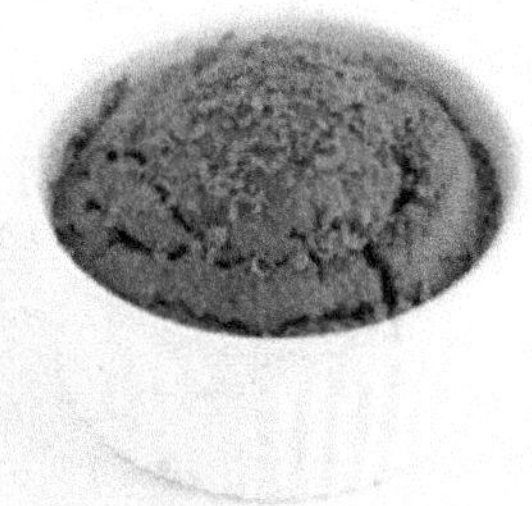 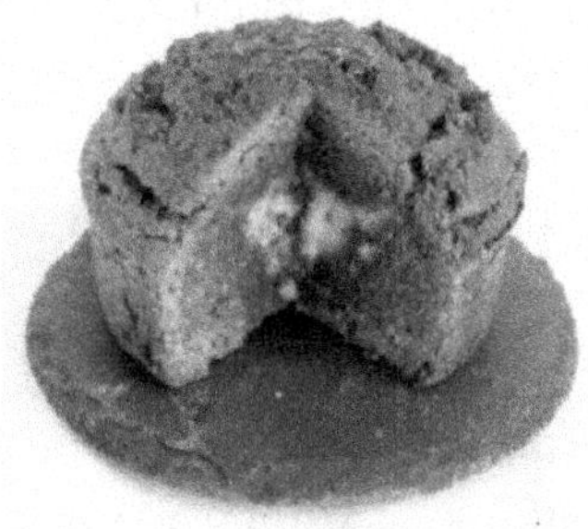

Ingredients:

6 tbs almond flour

2 tbs coconut flour

1 pinch coarse salt

7,1 oz (200 g) 85% chocolate

3,5 oz (100 g) sweet butter

2 tbs coconut oil

4 eggs

1,4 oz (40 g) sweetener stevia and erythritol blend for my part

1 tsp baking powder

1/2 tsp xanthan gum optional

1,8 oz (50 g) salted roasted peanuts

The preparation:

- In a bowl, mix the flours, yeast, coarse salt, sweetener and xanthan gum

- Add the eggs one by one, beating with an electric whisk

- Melt the butter, coconut oil and chocolate in a bain-marie or microwave

- Add the melted chocolate and butter mixture to the dough and mix until a homogeneous dough is obtained

- Spread in a baking dish and sprinkle with the previously crushed peanuts.

- Bake at 356 ° F (180 ° C) between 20 and 30 minutes depending on the size and shape of the mold.

CINNAMON STARS

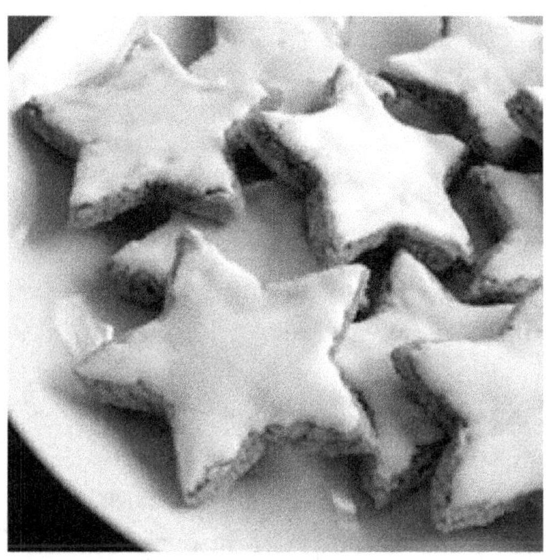

Ingredients:

14,1 oz (400 g) almond powder

3 egg whites

7,1 oz (200 g) erythritol powder

1 tsp lemon juice

1 tsp ground cinnamon

The preparation:

- Preheat the oven to 300 ° F (150 ° C)

- Beat the egg whites

- Add the erythritol and lemon juice and continue to whisk until everything is mixed

- Add the almond powder and cinnamon. Work the mixture to make a paste

- Cover the dough and put in the fridge for an hour

- Place the dough on a piece of baking paper, then cover with another piece. Roll about 1 cm thick

- Cut out the stars with a cookie cutter

- Place the cookies on a baking sheet lined with baking paper and bake for about 18 minutes (check the cooking from 12-14 minutes)

I hope you liked the book and enjoyed the recipes. It means a lot to me if you found this book helpful and I would like to hear about it. If you would like to leave a review, it will be highly appreciated and I like to hear from you.

Thank you very much for reading my book and I sincerely hope it helped you on your keto journey!

Logan